Cannabis Gourmet

A Simply Cannabis Cookbook to Learn the
Art of Cooking with Weed.

Jeff Sorensen

Table of Contents

1. Marijuana Lollipop

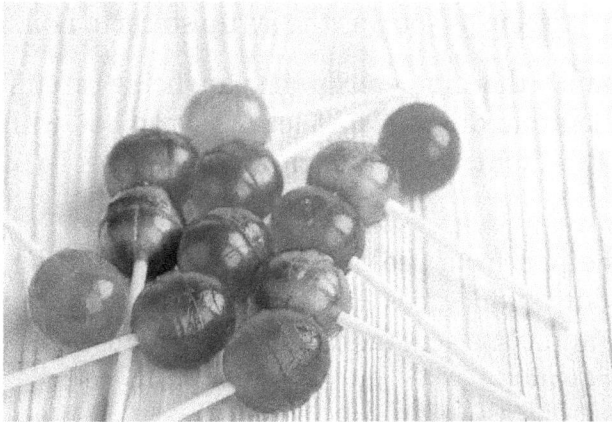

Ingredients:

1 cup sugar

1/3 cup corn syrup 1/2 cup water

1/4 teaspoon cream of tartar 1/4 to 1 teaspoon flavoring Liquid food coloring

1 or 2 teaspoon(s) citric acid (optional) 3 tablespoons cannabis tincture

Directions:

1.   Prepare either a marble slab or an upside-down cookie sheet (air underneath the sheet will help the candy to cool faster) by covering it with parchment paper and spraying it with oil. If you're using molds, prepare the molds with lollipop sticks, spray with oil, and place them on a cookie sheet or marble slab.

2.   In your pan, over medium heat, stir together the sugar, corn syrup, water and cream of tartar with a wooden spoon until the sugar crystals dissolve.

3.   Continue to stir, using a pastry brush dampened with warm water to dissolve any sugar crystals clinging to the sides of the pan, then stop stirring as soon as the syrup starts to boil.

4.   Place the candy thermometer in the pan, being careful not to let it touch the bottom or sides, and let the syrup boil without stirring until the thermometer just reaches 300 degrees F (hard-crack stage).

5.   Remove the pan from the heat immediately, and let the syrup cool to about 275 degrees F before adding flavor, color, cannabis tincture and citric acid (adding it sooner causes most of the flavor to cook away).

Caution

Be careful! The sugar syrup is extremely hot! If you burn yourself, run cold water over your hand for several minutes, but do not apply ice.

1.   Working quickly, pour the syrup into the prepared molds and let cool for about 10 minutes. If you're not using molds, pour small (2-inch) circles onto the prepared marble slab or cookie sheet, and place a lollipop stick in each one, twisting the stick to be sure it's covered with candy.

2.   Let the lollipops cool for at least 10 minutes, until they are hard. Wrap individually in plastic wrap or cellophane and seal with tape or twist ties.

3.   Store in a cool, dry place.

2. Marijuana Toffee Candy

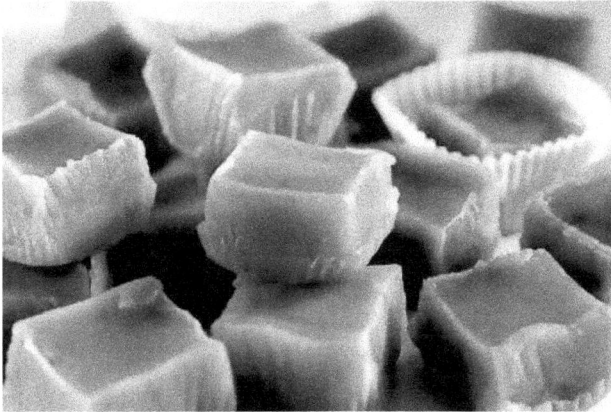

This recipe will introduce you to toffee, and from here you can experiment with adding nuts or other flavorings.

Ingredients:

2   cups roasted nuts (I like pecans) 1 cup sugar

1 cup butter (or cannabutter) 1 tablespoon light corn syrup 1/4 cup water

1 cup chocolate morsels

Directions:

1.   Spread about 1 1/2 cups of chopped nuts on a non-stick baking sheet (may need to lightly grease it, but not too much).

2.   Bring sugar, butter and corn syrup to a boil over medium heat, stirring constantly to prevent burning.

3.   Cook until the mixture reads about 300 to 310 degrees and mixture is golden brown (use candy thermometer and work fast; once it reaches 300, there isn't a lot of time until it burns).

4.   Pour sugar mixture over chopped nuts on the baking sheet. Spread chocolate over hot candy and spread with a spoon (chocolate will start melting as soon as it hits the candy).

5. Sprinkle the rest of the nuts over the top of the chocolate, and let the sheet cool for about 30 mins or until the candy is cool.

6. The candy should break apart pretty easily after it has cooled.

3. Cannabis Peanut Butter Balls

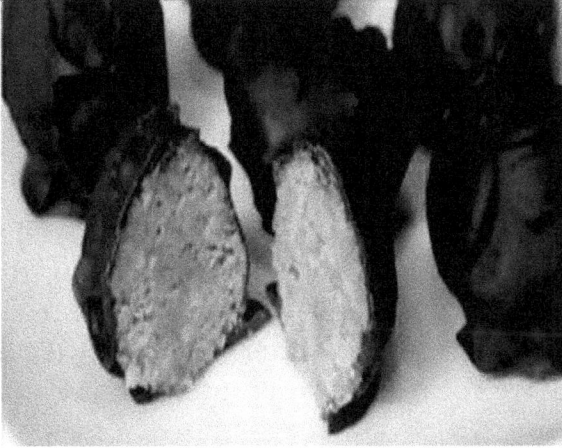

Items Needed:

Mixing bowl Double boiler Tray

Wax paper Toothpicks

Ingredients:

1 1/2 cups peanut butter

1 cup cannabutter (hardened) 4 cups confectioners' sugar

1 1/3 cups Graham cracker crumbs 2 cups semisweet chocolate chips 1 tablespoon shortening

Directions:

1.   Place the peanut butter and the cannabutter in a large mixing bowl. Slowly blend in the confectioners' sugar making sure that it does not get messy. Add Graham cracker crumbs and mix till consistency becomes solid enough to shape into balls. Make one-inch diameter balls.

2.   Melt the chocolate chips and shortening in a double bottomed boiler. Prick a toothpick into each ball, and then dip them one by one in the chocolate mixture. Place the chocolate wrapped balls on wax paper on a tray. Place in the freezer for about 30 minutes until the balls are all solid.

3.   This is an easy way to have a sweet snack and a cannabis kick at the same time. Just don't gobble them all down at once; go gradually, savor them, and relish them like you really want to. Share these awesome peanut butter balls with your friends, so that you all can feel the mellow kick coming on slowly, sweetly but surely!

4. Rice Krispie Treats

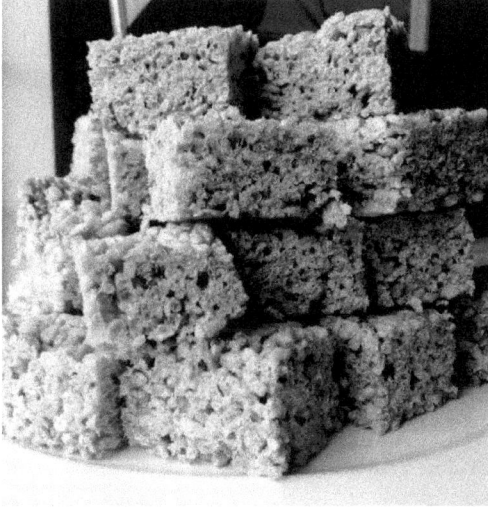

Making a good batch of weed-infused Rice Crispy treats comes down to using high-quality ingredients and following a few simple directions. Use this helpful step-by-step guide to get started with your first batch of canna- crispies.

Ingredients:

1   bag miniature marshmallows (use fruit flavored marshmallows to change it up)

2   tablespoons unsalted butter (cannabis-infused butter) 2 tablespoons coconut oil (cannabis-infused coconut oil) 5 cups crispy rice cereal

¼ teaspoon almond extract (try a raspberry or strawberry with fruit flavored marshmallows)

Note: You can choose to use both infused butter and coconut oil or just use one or the other.

Directions:

1.   Spray bottom of cookie sheet with cooking spray (or parchment paper makes easier cleanup).

2.   In pan over medium heat, melt butter, infused oil and extract together.

3.   Continue heating over medium heat, and slowly add marshmallows to the mixture, stirring constantly to prevent scorching.

4.   When the mixture is well-blended (remember don't overcook), remove from heat and immediately add cereal in small portions until the cereal is evenly covered. (Tip: Coat your spoon with a little oil first.)

5.   Spread out onto cookie sheet, and press down with spoon into desired thickness.

6.   Allow to cool and then cut into individual portions (15-20 servings).

7.   Chocolate lovers can drizzle canna-shell chocolate across the top before cooling.

Caution

1.   Too Much Caffeine Can Negatively Affect Your Experience:

2.   If using chocolate in your recipe, please consider that caffeine is found naturally in cocoa beans, so any chocolate has a little bit of the stimulant. Candy bars generally have less than 10 milligrams, but the darker the chocolate, the higher the caffeine content.

5. Cannabis Apple Pie

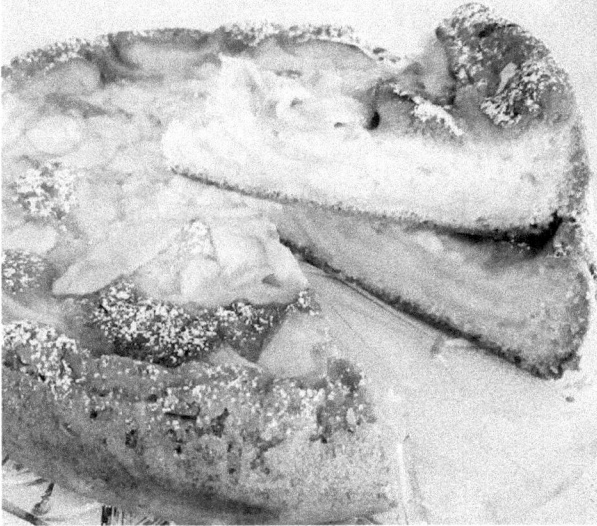

Time Required: 2 Hours

Ingredients:

9-inch pie dish

2 sheets of refrigerated pie crusts

6 cups apples, cored, peeled, and sliced (Granny Smith, Golden Delicious, and/or HoneyCrisp)

1 tablespoon fresh lemon juice

⅓ cup brown sugar

½ cup granulated sugar

⅛ cup flour

1   teaspoon cinnamon, ground

½ teaspoon salt

⅛ teaspoon nutmeg, ground 1½ cups cannabutter, cubed

Directions :

1.   Preheat oven to 375 degrees.

2.   Press one pie crust sheet firmly into the bottom of the pie dish and up the sides of the pan.

3.   Trim the edge of the dough with kitchen scissors; leave 1 inch of dough to hang over the edge of pan. Set aside.

4.   Combine the apples and lemon juice in a large bowl. Mix well.

5.   Add brown sugar, granulated sugar, flour, cinnamon, salt and nutmeg.

6.   Mix well, making sure to coat all the apples.

7.   Transfer the filling mix to the dough-lined pan.

8.   Disperse cubed cannabutter on top of the apple filling evenly.

9.   Place the second pie sheet over the filled pie. Trim edges appropriately, leaving 1 inch of dough hanging.

10.   Fold the edge of the top layer of dough under the edge of the bottom layer of dough. Pinch dough sheets together to seal.

11.   Cut an "x" across the top center of the dough to allow steam to escape.

12.   Put the uncooked pie in the refrigerator to firm the dough (about 20 minutes).

13.   Remove pie from refrigerator and bake the pie in the preheated oven for 1 hour, or until the crust is golden brown and the filling is bubbling.

14.   Transfer pie to a wire rack and let cool to completely set for at least 1 hour before serving.

15. Serve with whipped canna-cream or cannabis ice cream for a heightened experience!

6. Cannabis-Infused Red Velvet Cake

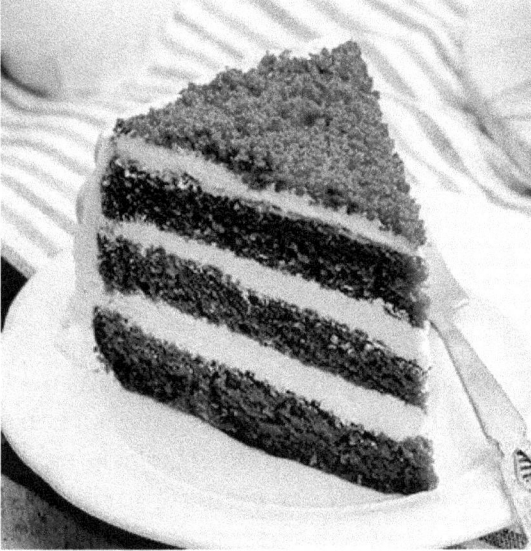

Red velvet cake always elicits wows from guests, probably because of its dramatic look, and these cupcakes, kicked up with ganja, are no exception.

Ingredients:

2   3/4 cups all purpose flour 1 3/4 cups sugar

1   teaspoon baking soda

2   teaspoons cocoa powder

2 large eggs, room temperature

¾ cannabis oil (coconut, canola…)

¾ cup canola oil

1   1/4 cup buttermilk

2   teaspoons red food coloring 1 teaspoon vanilla

1 tablespoon white vinegar

For Frosting:

16 ounces cream cheese

4 ounces cannabis butter, slightly softened 3 cups powdered sugar

2 teaspoons vanilla

Directions:

This cake is so very good; you will love having it in your repertoire. When you eat a slice that is medicated, be sure to save another sliver for later. It's one of those foods that you eat when you are stoned and want to just sit there eating it for the rest of your life. Fortunately, that feeling will pass, as it would not be a very productive, though delicious, experience.

1.   Preheat oven to 325 degrees F.

2.   Place parchment on the bottom of three 8-inch pans.

3.   Mix all dry ingredients together. Beat eggs slightly. Add all wet ingredients together. Mix wet into dry ingredients.

4.   Pour into prepared pans. Bake for 30 to 35 minutes.

5.   When done, remove from oven and wait 5 minutes; then, turn out on cooling racks

For Icing:

1.   Place the butter in mixer and beat till soft. Add cream cheese and mix, stopping periodically to scrape bowl.

2.   Beat till light colored; slowly add powdered sugar, waiting for it to be completely incorporated along with some air before adding more.

3.   When all the sugar is incorporated, beat a few more minutes; add vanilla, beat and ice cake immediately.

7. Peanut Butter Ganja Goo Balls

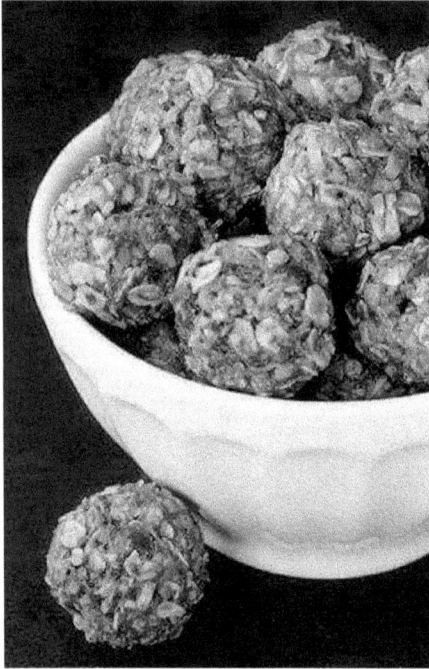

Yield: 15 Ganja Goo Balls

If you are planning to make a homemade edible, the general process is relatively simple. This particular recipe is for your very own Ganja Goo- Balls.

N.B. The following recipe is made with an estimated amount of marijuana. Remember that edibles can hit harder than you expect, so feel free to judge the amounts according to your own experience. It is strongly advised to first learn how to calculate the strength of edibles.

Ingredients:

250 g melted cannabutter 225 g oats

250 g peanut butter (whether it is the smooth or chunky variant will be all up to you)

3 tablespoon honey

2 tablespoon ground cinnamon 1-2 tablespoon cocoa powder

Directions:

1.   Place all ingredients in one large bowl and stir until everything is mixed in.

2.   Place the mix into the freezer and leave it for 10-20 minutes.

Mold the mixture into individual balls, to the size of your preference. After which, drop it onto some wax paper to set. Some people prefer adding other

ingredients such as chopped walnuts, raisins, Rice Krispies or Corn Flakes, just to experiment.

1.   More oats can be added if you find the end result a little too sticky and gooey, or add more honey or peanut butter if it turns out to be too dry. It is all about being creative and adding your own touch to this delicacy.

2.   Once that is done, you are now ready to serve this scrumptious treat, which can be eaten for dessert, a snack, or just any time of the day you choose to have an edible. Enjoy!

8. Cannabis Monkey Bread

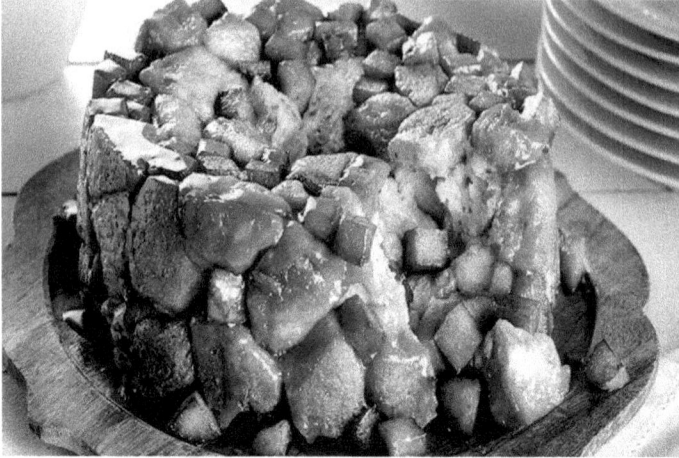

Yield: 4-6 Servings

If you've never had the privilege of eating monkey bread, look no further! The missing link to your happiness is here. Monkey bread is a fun, rip-apart bread, dripping in buttery and sugary goodness. This recipe is extremely simple to make, and generously feeds a good amount of people, making this a perfect breakfast dish.

Ingredients:

2   cans of original home-style pre-packaged biscuits (not the flaky-layers 1 cup sugar

2 oranges, zested

1 teaspoon cinnamon A pinch of salt

1 cup light brown sugar 1 stick of butter

1 stick of cannabutter

1   tablespoon organic pure vanilla extract

Directions:

1.   Preheat oven to 350 degrees F. Leave 2 cans of biscuits in the refrigerator until you plan on using them – the colder the biscuits, the less likely they will stick together during the sugar-coating process.

2.   Add the white sugar, orange zest, cinnamon and a pinch of salt to a gallon-size, re-sealable plastic bag.

3.   Once your sugar bag is ready, you may remove the two cans of biscuits from the refrigerator and open them. Using a pair of kitchen scissors, cut each biscuit into quarters. After cutting roughly 3-4 biscuits, add the pieces to the plastic bag, seal it, and shake the bag around until all the pieces are covered in the sugar/orange zest blend.

4.   It is recommended that you add batches of 3 - 4 biscuits to the sugar bag at a time, as this will help prevent the pieces from clumping together into one big ball of dough. Repeat this process until both cans of biscuits are quartered, tossed in the sugar bag and evenly coated.

5.   Generously spray your bundt pan with some non-stick baking spray, making sure to cover every nook and crevice.

6.   Pour the contents of the bag evenly into your bundt pan, rearranging some pieces of biscuit, if need be. Set the bundt pan to the side for now.

7.   In a medium skillet, heat your butter and cannabutter over medium to medium-low heat, until just about fully melted – do not burn the butter. Add in your light brown sugar and vanilla extract, and stir until almost thoroughly combined. It's okay if there are some small chunks of brown sugar still in the butter.

8.   Then, carefully pour your butter/sugar mixture over the chunks of biscuit, turning the bundt pan as you pour to ensure even coverage. Shimmy the pan when you're done to make sure all the butter and sugar finds its way to the bottom of the pan.

9.   Pop the bundt pan in the oven for 35-40 minutes, checking often towards the end of the cook time. No spaces in between bits of biscuit chunks should appear doughy, and the top of the monkey bread will have a delicious golden brown color.

10.   Remove the bundt pan from the oven and onto a cooling rack for 10 minutes and WAIT! This is the most difficult part!

11.   You need to allow the buttery, caramel sauce to cool enough so that when you flip over the bundt cake pan, the sauce does not drip all over and create a huge mess.

12.   After 10 minutes, carefully flip and transfer your monkey bread to a large platter. Be careful as the bread will be extremely hot!

13.   Serve and enjoy!

9. Cannabis Cinnamon Roll Oatmeal Cookie

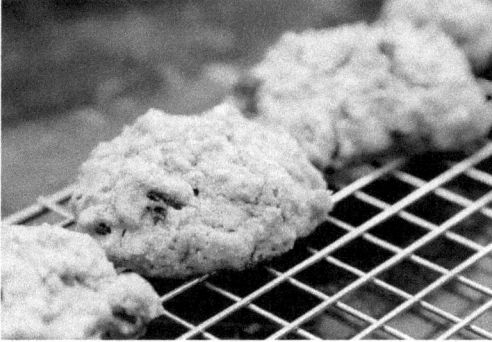

Ingredients:

10 packets cinnamon roll instant oatmeal 1 cup of firmly packed brown sugar

1 teaspoon baking soda 2 eggs

1 cup softened cannabutter 2 cups all-purpose flour

3/4 cup white sugar 1/4 cup of water

Directions:

1.   Preheat your oven to 350 degrees F.

2.   Mix butter and the sugars together until they're a creamy consistency.

3.   Take the two eggs and beat them in. Then, add in both the flour and the baking soda, stirring continuously. Then, add in all of the oatmeal packets as well as the 1/4 cup of water.

4.   Stir everything together until mixed evenly. The mixture should be like cookie dough.

5.   Make small round balls out of the dough, and place on a greased cookie sheet.

6.   Bake them in the oven for about 12 minutes, until they are golden brown. Remove the cookies from the sheet immediately, and put them on a plate to cool off before enjoying!

10. Carrot Cakecannabis

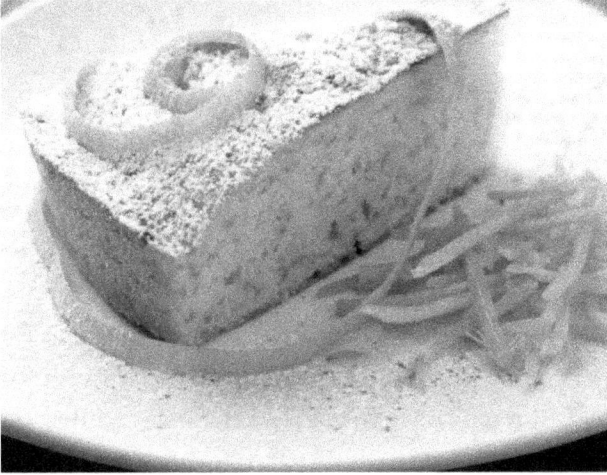

Serves: 18

Ingredients:

4 eggs

1   1/4 cups vegetable oil 2 cups white sugar

2   teaspoons vanilla extract 2 cups all-purpose flour

2 teaspoons baking soda

2 teaspoons baking powder 1/2 teaspoon salt

2 teaspoons ground cinnamon 3 cups grated carrots

1 cup chopped pecans

For Frosting:

1/4 cup marijuana butter

¼ cup vegetable oil

8 ounces cream cheese, softened 4 cups confectioners' sugar

1 teaspoon vanilla extract 1 cup chopped pecans

Directions:

1.   Preheat oven to 350 degrees F.

2.   Grease and flour a 9×13 inch pan. In a large bowl, beat together eggs, oil, white sugar and 2 teaspoons vanilla. Mix in flour, baking soda, baking powder, salt and cinnamon. Stir in carrots. Fold in pecans.

3.   Pour into prepared pan. Bake in the preheated oven for 40 to 50 minutes, or until a toothpick inserted into the center of the cake comes out clean. Let cool in pan for 10 minutes, then turn out onto a wire rack and cool completely.

For Frosting:

1.   In a medium bowl, combine both butters, cream cheese, confectioners' sugar and 1 teaspoon vanilla. Beat until the mixture is smooth and creamy. Stir in chopped pecans. Frost the cooled cake.

11. Chocolate Cakecannabis

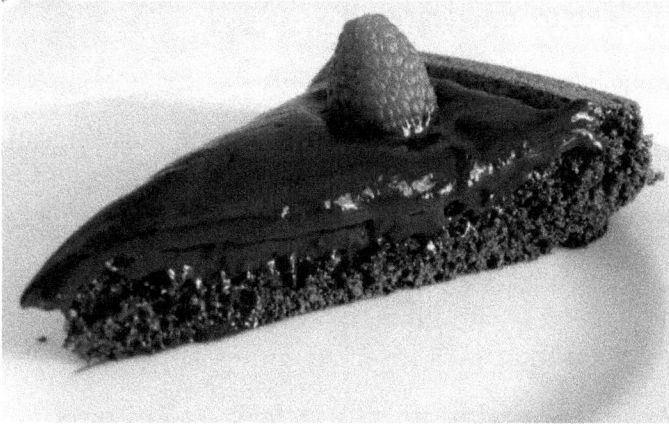

Serves: 12

Ingredients:

1 (18.25 ounce) package Devil's food cake mix

1   (5.9 ounce) package instant chocolate pudding mix 1 cup sour cream

1/4 cup marijuana oil

¾ cup vegetable oil 4 eggs

1/2 cup warm water

2   cups semisweet chocolate chips

Directions:

1.   Preheat oven to 350 degrees F.

2.   In a large bowl, mix together the cake and pudding mixes, sour cream, marijuana oil, vegetable oil, beaten eggs and water. Stir in the chocolate chips and pour batter into a well-greased 12 cup bundt pan.

3.   Bake for 50 to 55 minutes, or until top is springy to the touch and a wooden toothpick inserted comes out clean.

4.   Cool cake thoroughly in pan at least 1 ½ hours before inverting onto a plate. If desired, dust the cake with powdered sugar.

12. Chocolate Brownie Cakecannabis

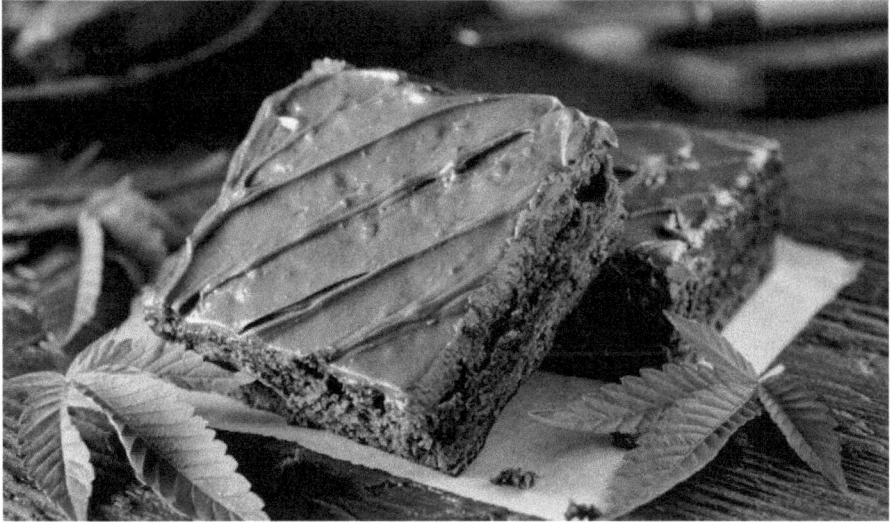

Serves: 12

Ingredients:

1 (18.25 ounce) package Devil's food cake mix

1 (3.9 ounce) package instant chocolate pudding mix 4 eggs

1   cup sour cream

1/4 cup marijuana oil

¼ cup vegetable oil

½ cup water

2   cups semisweet chocolate chips

Directions:

1.   Preheat oven to 350 degrees F.

2.   Grease and flour a 10-inch Bundt pan.

3.   Be sure all ingredients are at room temperature. In a large bowl, stir together cake mix and pudding mix.

4.   Make a well in the center and pour in eggs, sour cream, marijuana oil, vegetable oil and water.

5.   Beat on low speed until blended. Scrape bowl, and beat 4 minutes on medium speed. Stir in chocolate chips.

6.   Pour batter into prepared pan. Bake in oven for 50 to 60 minutes, or until a toothpick inserted into the center of the cake comes out clean. Allow to cool before serving.

13. Coconut Cakecannabis

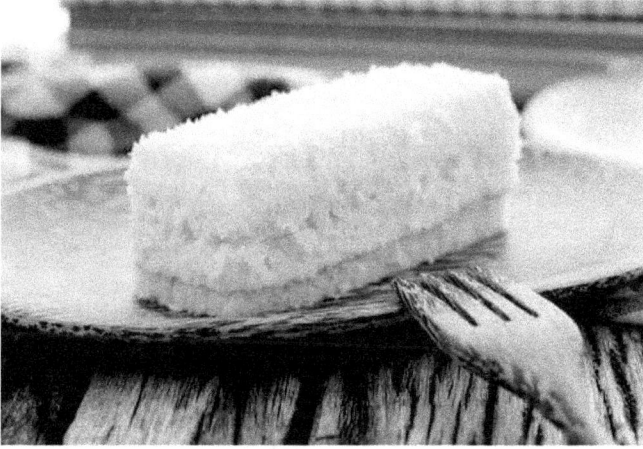

Serves: 24

Ingredients:

1 (18.25 ounce) package yellow cake mix

1 (3.5 ounce) package instant vanilla pudding mix 1 1/3 cups water

4 eggs

1/4 cup marijuana oil 2 cups flaked coconut

1 cup chopped walnuts

4 tablespoons butter, melted 2 cups flaked coconut

2 teaspoons milk

1/2 teaspoon vanilla extract

1 (8 ounce) package cream cheese 3 1/2 cups confectioners' sugar

Directions:

1.	Preheat oven to 350 degrees F. Grease a 9×13 inch pan. In a large bowl, combine cake mix, pudding mix, water, eggs and marijuana oil. Blend for 4 minutes. Stir in 2 cups coconut and the chopped nuts. Pour into a greased 9×13 inch pan.

2.	Bake for 30 minutes or until done. Allow to cool.

For Frosting:

1.	Melt 2 tablespoons of butter over low heat. Add 3/4 cup of the coconut and stir until browned.

2.	Dry on paper towel. Cream other 2 tablespoons butter with cream cheese. Alternately add milk and powdered sugar. Add vanilla.

3.	Stir in remaining 1-1/4 cup coconut. Spread Icing on cake and sprinkle with browned coconut.

14. CBD Gummy Bears

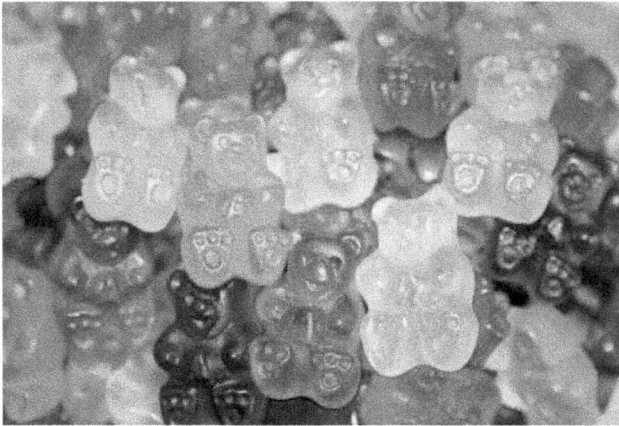

For this recipe, you can either make your own CBD oil or tincture. Once you have that ready, all you need is a gummy bear mold and a couple of ingredients.

Ingredients:

300mg CBD oil or tincture

1 package of JELLO (3 oz size) 1 tablespoon of gelatin

1/2 cup of water Gummy bear molds

Directions:

1.   Pour 1/2 cup of water into a sauce pan set on low heat.

2.   Add 1 package of Jello (3 oz size).

3.   Add 1 tablespoon of gelatin.

4.   Mix until dissolved and then remove from heat.

5.   While still hot, add your CBD tincture/oil and whisk well.

6.   Using the dropper, add into your mold.

15. True Belgian Cannabis Waffles

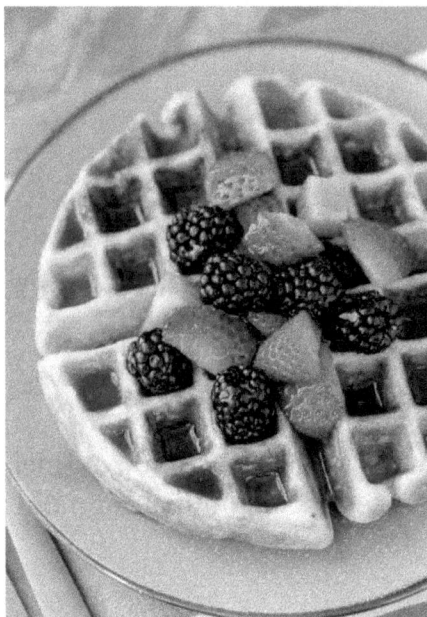

This homemade cannabis Belgian waffle recipe is easy and makes delicious Belgian waffles with a twist of cannabutter! These waffles are perfectly crisp and golden on the outside while being light and fluffy on the inside!

Ingredients:

1/4 cup cannabis butter 2 cups all-purpose flour 3/4 cup sugar

3-1/2 teaspoons baking powder 2 large eggs, separated

1-1/2 cups whole milk 1 cup butter, melted

1 teaspoon vanilla extract

Sliced fresh strawberries or syrup

Directions:

1.   In a bowl, combine flour, sugar and baking powder.

2.   In another bowl, lightly beat egg yolks. Add milk, butter, cannabis butter and vanilla; mix well. Stir into dry ingredients just until combined.

3.   Beat egg whites until stiff peaks form; fold into batter.

4.   Bake in a preheated waffle iron according to manufacturer's directions until golden brown.

5.   Serve with strawberries or syrup.

16. Cannabis Easter Egg

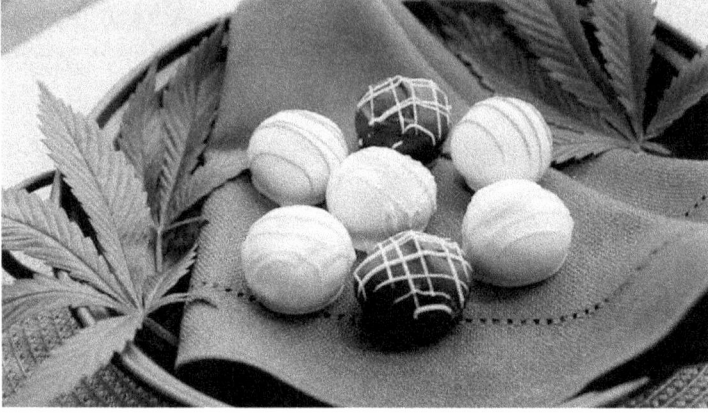

Ingredients:

1/4 cup cannabis butter

1 cup chocolate (70% cocoa solids) or milk chocolate.

Directions:

1.   In a large bowl, mix your chocolate and cannabis butter.

2.   Half-fill a small pan with water and bring to a gentle simmer over a low heat. Rest your bowl with chocolate on top, then allow to melt, stirring occasionally.

3.   Using oven gloves, remove the bowl from the heat and leave to cool to 95 degrees F (35°C). Check the temperature with a cooking thermometer.

4.   Spoon the chocolate into your mold, one tablespoon at a time, tilting the mold so the chocolate covers the surface. Don't worry if you make a mess! Tip any excess chocolate back into the bowl.

5.   Allow the chocolate to cool slightly, then, using a butter knife, scrape around the rim of the mold to get a clean edge.

6.   Meanwhile, repeat steps 4 to 6 with the second mold.

7.   Lay out some greaseproof paper and place the mold flat-side-down on top for 15 minutes or until the chocolate has completely set.

8.   To remove your eggs from their molds, squeeze the casing gently, working your way around the edge (the warmth from your hands will help).

9.   Brush the remaining melted chocolate around the rim of each of the chocolate egg halves, then gently press them together so they stick in place. Leave for a few minutes until the chocolate sets, then it's ready!

17.Weed-Infused Sugar Cookie Christmas Tree

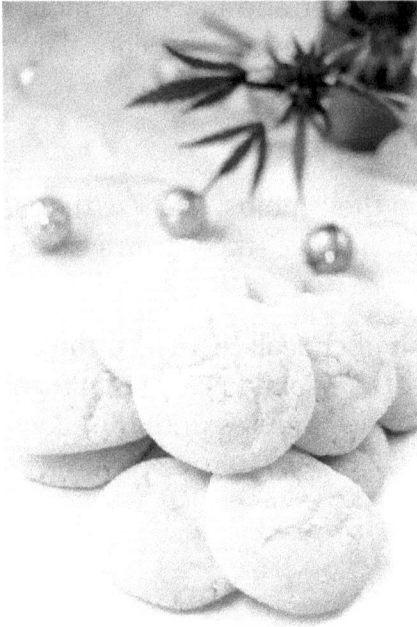

Ingredients:

3/4 cup unsalted butter, room temperature 1/4 cup cannabis butter, room temperature 1 cup sugar

1   large egg, room temperature 1 teaspoon pure vanilla extract 1/2 teaspoon almond extract

2   teaspoon baking powder 2 1/2 cups all-purpose flour 1/2 cup cocoa powder

For Buttercream:

1/2 cup unsalted butter, room temperature 1/4 cup cannabis sugar

1 teaspoon vanilla extract

1/2 teaspoon pure almond extract 3 cups confectioners' sugar, sifted

1 -2 tablespoons whole milk, you can use more if needed Green food color

Pinch salt

Directions:

For Cookies:

1.   Preheat oven to 350 degrees F.

2.   Add both butters to the bowl of your stand mixer and cream on medium- high for 1-2 minutes, or until butter is smooth.

3.   With the mixer on low, slowly add the sugar and then the egg.

4.   Scrape the bowl with the mixer off.

5.   Turn mixer back on low and add in extracts.

6.   Allow all ingredients to combine fully.

7.   Add the baking powder and then the flour, 1/2 cup at a time, until fully incorporated; ending with the cocoa powder.

8.   Remove bowl from mixer and drop dough onto a floured countertop. Roll out into a flat disc, about 1/2 inch thick.

9.   Cut cookies into 2-inch, 1 1/2-inch, and 1-inch cookies and bake for 6-9 minutes.

10.   Let cool on the cookie sheet until firm enough to transfer to a cooling rack.

For Buttercream:

1.   Beat butter together with cannabis sugar in the bowl of stand mixer with paddle attachment on medium-high speed until light and fluffy (about 3 minutes).

2.   With the mixer off or on low, add vanilla and almond extract.

3.   Slowly add in confectioners' sugar, cannabis sugar, milk, green food color and salt; frequently scrape sides and bottom of the bowl.

4.   Once incorporated, whip frosting for at least 3 minutes on medium-high to high.

5.   If frosting is too thick to spread, gradually beat in additional milk.

6.   Store in refrigerator up to 2 weeks. Rewhip before using.

18. Weed Donuts

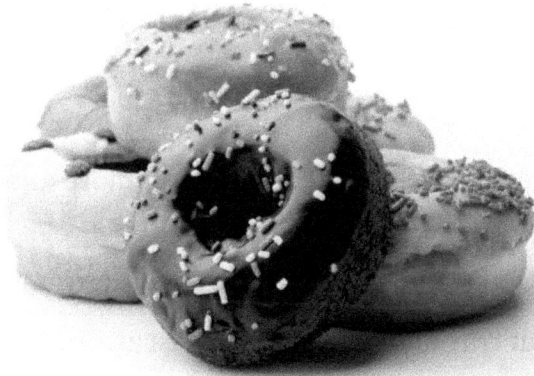

Ingredients:

1 1/2 cups cannabis sugar 3/4 cup lukewarm milk

1 envelope yeast

1 tablespoon sugar

1   egg

1/4 cup melted butter 1/3 cup sugar

2   1/2 cups flour 1/2 teaspoon salt

Directions:

1.   In a medium bowl, add milk, 1 tablespoon sugar and yeast. Whisk and set aside.

2.   In another bowl, add 1 egg, 1/3 cup sugar, melted butter and whisk.

3.   Add yeast mixture to the egg mixture and whisk well.

4.   In a large bowl, add flour, salt and wet mixture; mix and knead until smooth and no longer sticky.

5.   Move the dough to a greased bowl and cover; set aside until it has doubled in size.

6.   When doubled in size, knead dough once more and flatten out on a surface using a bread roller.

7.   Cut donut-sized rounds in the dough using a round cutter.

8.   Place on a flat tray and let double in size again.

9.   Now fry your donuts for 2 minutes each side in vegetable oil on 350 degrees F.

10.   Coat with cannabis sugar straight after frying.

11.   Fill donuts with jelly or nutella.

19.Homemade Cannabis Oreo Cookies

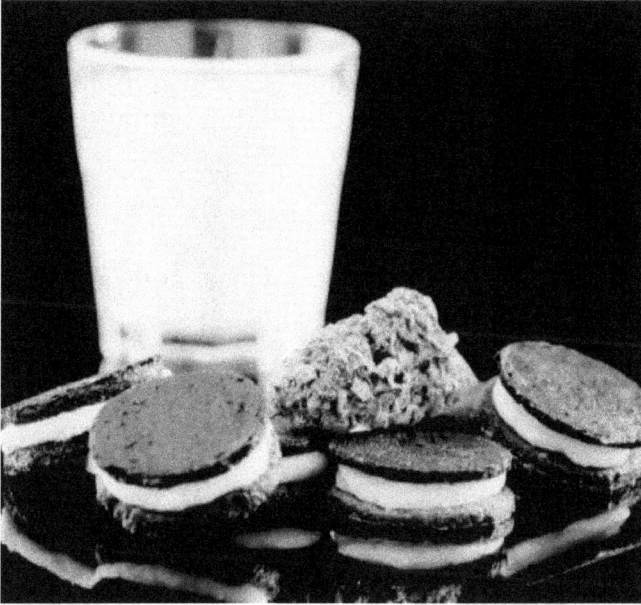

Ingredients:

1   cup 50/50 butter/cannabis butter mixed 1 cup sugar

2   teaspoons salt

2 large eggs

2 cups all-purpose flour

1 ¼ cups dark cocoa powder

½ teaspoon baking soda

For Cream Filling:

½ cup cannabis butter 2 cups powdered sugar 1 teaspoon vanilla

Directions:

1.   Preheat oven to 325 degrees F .

2.   In a large bowl, cream together 1/2 cup cannabis butter with ½ cup normal butter. Mix with the white sugar and salt until light and fluffy.

3.   Beat in eggs until fully incorporated.

4.   Sieve together the flour, cocoa powder, and baking soda into the mix. Blend well.

5.   Add the dry ingredients to the wet ingredients, and mix together until combined.

6.   Turn the dough out onto your surface and push together into a flat square. Wrap the dough in plastic wrap and refrigerate for 1 hour.

For Cream Filling:

1.   To make the filling, combine ½ cup cannabis butter, powdered sugar, and vanilla in a medium mixing bowl. Beat together until light and fluffy.

2.   Remove the dough from the fridge, and for ease of rolling out, divide the dough into 4 pieces.

3.   To roll out the dough, place a quarter of the dough between two sheets of parchment paper. Roll the dough between the two sheets of parchment to

¼-inch thickness.

4.   Using a small round cookie cutter or champagne glass, cut the dough into individual rounds and place on a large parchment-lined baking sheet, leaving at least ½-inch between each cookie.

5. Pack together and re-roll out any scraps to cut additional cookies. Repeat this process with each remaining ¼ of the dough.

6. Bake in preheated oven for 15 minutes.

7. Remove and transfer cookies to a cooling rack to cool completely.

8. Assemble the cookies by spreading a generous scoop of the icing onto one of the cookies and sandwiching it with another. Give it a light squeeze and scrape any excess off to clear and even out the sides.

9. Serve with a glass of milk.

20. Cannabis Chocolate Caramel Peanut Butter Cups

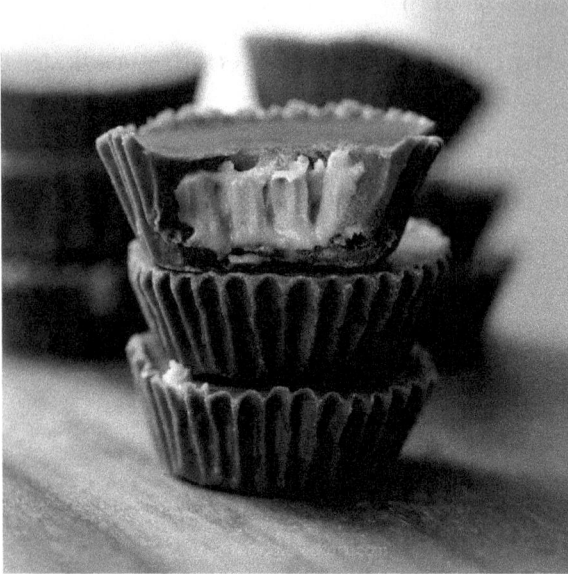

There are so many cannabis chocolate desserts that are a treat, but this must top all of them.

Ingredients:

4 tablespoons cannabis butter 2 1/2 cups chocolate

1/2 cup salted caramel sauce 1 cup peanut butter

1/2 cup powdered sugar 1/4 cup cornflakes Pinch of salt

Directions:

1.   Take a medium bowl and melt chocolate au bain marie with your cannabis butter.

2.   Mix using a spatula so your cannabis butter is evenly mixed into the chocolate.

3.   Put your chocolate cannabis mix in a piping bag and let cool slightly.

4.   Line up a tray with 12 paper cupcake cups.

5.   Use half of your chocolate cannabis mix to fill out the cups evenly. A thin layer just so the bottom is covered will do.

6.   Freeze for 5 minutes until chocolate is solid.

7.   Add a good tablespoon of caramel sauce to each chocolate cup.

8.   Freeze again for 5 minutes

9.   In a medium small bowl, mix 1 cup peanut butter with the cornflakes, powdered sugar and cannabis butter using a hand mixer.

10.   Add a full tablespoon of peanut butter to your chocolate cups.

11.   Now use the other half of your cannabis chocolate to cover the peanut butter.

12.   Freeze for about 15 - 20 minutes.

13.   Serve.

21. Cannabis-Infused Ice Cream

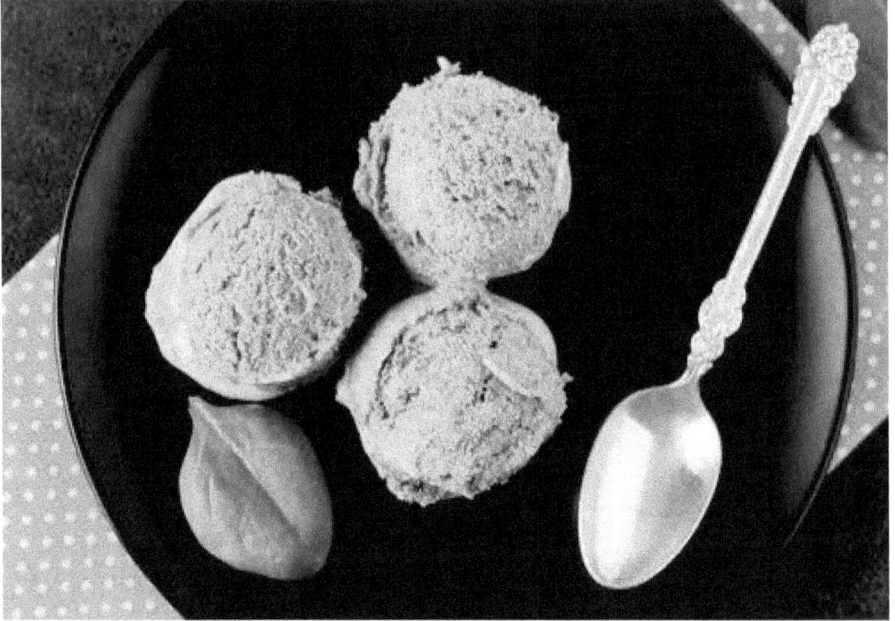

Cannabis-infused ice cream without an ice cream machine...perfect for a summer day.

Ingredients:

4 tablespoons cannabis butter 2 cups whipping cream

1 can (14oz) condensed milk 1/2 teaspoon vanilla extract 1/4 cup chopped mint

Directions:

1.   Whip the cream until stiff; add all remaining ingredients in separate bowl and mix.

2.   Now fold the mixture into the whipping cream. Store in a container and freeze for 6 hours.

3.   Serve the cannabis Ice cream.

22. Cannabis Pancakes

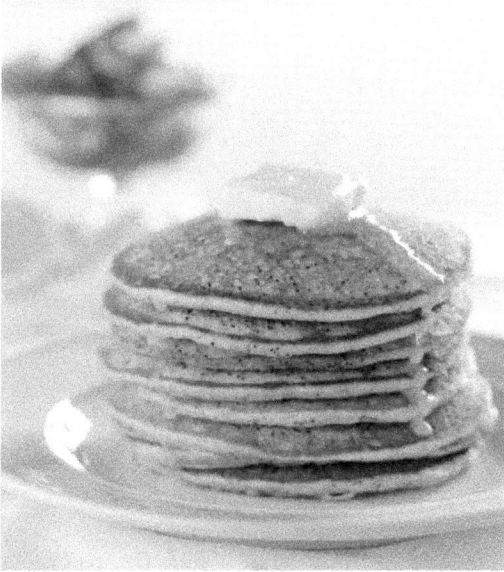

Ingredients:

1/2 cup cannabis milk 1/2 cup whole milk

1   cup all purpose flour

2   tablespoons white sugar 2 teaspoons baking powder 1 egg
beaten

2 tablespoons vegetable oil 1 teaspoon salt

Directions:

1.   In a large bowl, mix flour, sugar, baking powder and salt.
Make a well in the center, and pour in cannabis milk, whole milk,
egg and oil. Mix until smooth.

2.   Heat a lightly oiled griddle or frying pan over medium-high heat. Pour or scoop the batter onto the griddle, using approximately 1/4 cup for each pancake. Brown on both sides and serve hot.

3.   Serve the cannabis pancakes.

23. Marijuana Cheesecake

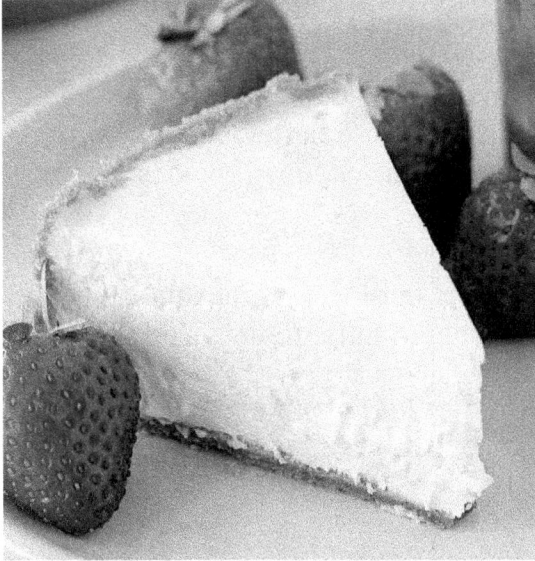

Ingredients:

2   tablespoons cannabis butter 1 tablespoon normal butter 24 oreo cookies, divided

3   (250 grams) Philadelphia cream cheese packets 3/4 cup sugar

1   teaspoon vanilla 3 eggs

Directions:

1.   Preheat oven to 330 degrees F.

2.   Place 16 of the cookies in resealable plastic bag. Flatten bag to remove excess air, then seal bag. Finely crush cookies by rolling a rolling pin across the bag.

3.   Place in bowl. Add butter; mix well. Press firmly onto bottom of 9-inch springform pan.

4.   Beat cream cheese, sugar and vanilla in large bowl with electric mixer on medium speed until well blended. Add eggs, 1 at a time, beating just until blended after each addition.

5.   Chop or crush remaining 8 cookies. Gently stir half of the chopped cookies into cream cheese batter. Pour over prepared crust; sprinkle with the remaining chopped cookies.

6.   Bake 45 minutes or until center is almost set. Cool. Refrigerate 3 hours or overnight. Cut into 12 pieces. Store leftover cheesecake in refrigerator.

7. Add Strawberry (if you want)

24. Cannabis Gingerbread

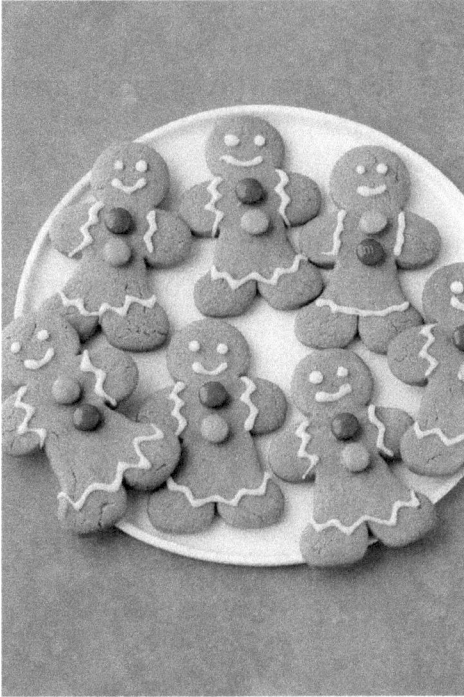

Ingredients:

1/4 cup cannabis butter 1/4 cup normal butter One egg

One cup molasses

2   1/2 cups all-purpose flour 1 1/2 teaspoons bakins soda 1 teaspoon ground cumin

1 teaspoon ground ginger 1/2 teaspoon salt

1 cup hot water

Directions:

1.   Preheat oven to 330 degrees F.

2.   Grease and flour a 9-inch square pan.

3. In a large bowl, cream together the sugar and butter. Beat in the egg, and mix in the molasses.

4. In a bowl, sift together the flour, baking soda, salt, cinnamon, ginger and cloves. Blend into the creamed mixture. Stir in the hot water. Pour into the prepared pan.

5. Bake 1 hour in the preheated oven until a knife inserted in the center comes out clean. Allow to cool in pan before serving.

25. Chocolate Cannabis Bar

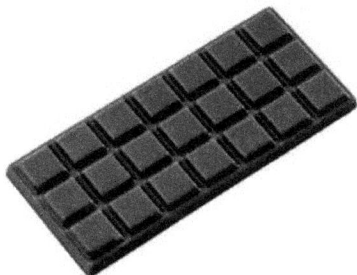

Ingredients:

1/4 cup cannabis butter 4 cups chocolate

Directions:

1.   Melt the chocolate in a clean, dry bowl set over a pan of barely simmering water. If you want to temper the chocolate, add your cannabis butter.

2.   Once the chocolate is melted (and tempered, if tempering the chocolate), remove the bowl from the pan and wipe the moisture off the bottom of the bowl.

3.   Pour or spoon a layer of chocolate into your molds. Rap them on the counter a few times to distribute the chocolate evenly and release any air bubbles; then working quickly, top with any kinds of nuts, dried fruits or other ingredients that you wish and press them in slightly.

4.   (You can also stir ingredients into the chocolate, such as toasted nuts, seeds, crisped rice cereal, snipped marshmallows or other ingredients, then pour the mixture into the molds.)

5. Immediately put the bars in the refrigerator until firm. If tempered chocolate is used, it shouldn't take more than five minutes for them to firmup. Otherwise, the chocolate will take longer.

26. Cannabis Muffins

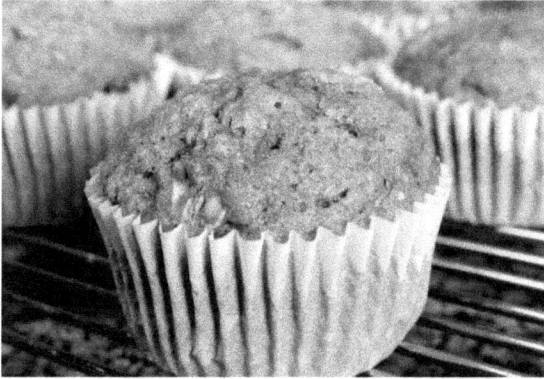

Ingredients:

1/4 cup melted cannabis butter 2 cups all-purpose flour

3 teaspoons baking powder 1/2 teaspoon salt

3/4 cup white sugar 1 egg

1 cup milk

Directions:

1.   Preheat oven to 350 degrees F.

2.   Melt cannabis butter on very low temperature.

3.   Stir together the flour, baking powder, salt and sugar in a large bowl. Make a well in the center. In a small bowl or 2 cup measuring cup, beat egg with a fork. Stir in milk and cannabis butter. Pour all at once into the well in the flour mixture.

4.   Mix quickly and lightly with a fork until moistened.The batter will be lumpy. Pour the batter into paper lined muffin pan cups.

5.   Bake for 25 minutes or until golden.

27. Chewy Chocolate Chip Weed Cookies

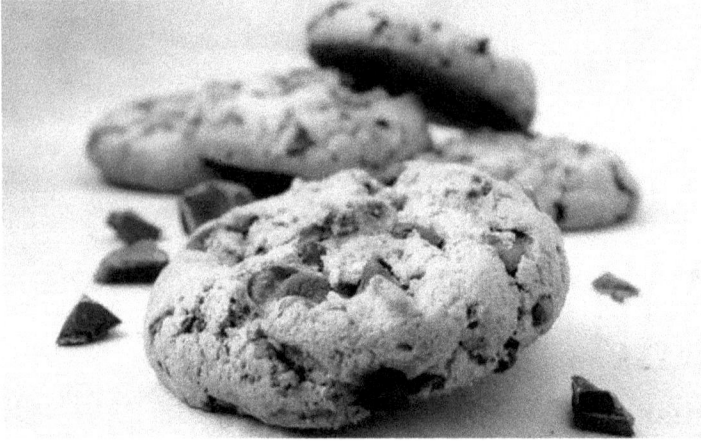

One cookie in the afternoon can help to make the rest of your work day bearable. One cannabis cookie is also a simple way to dose your medicinal cannabis before bed, and it helps soothe nighttime aches and pains.

Ingredients:

1/4 cup softened cannabis butter 1/2 cup softened normal butter 2 cups all-purpose flour

1/2 teaspoon baking soda 1/2 teaspoon salt

One cup brown sugar 1/2 cup white sugar

1 tablespoon vanilla extract 1 egg

1   egg yolk

2   cups chocolate chips

Directions:

1.   Preheat the oven to 325 degrees F.

2.   Grease cookie sheets or line with parchment paper.

3.   In a bowl, sift together the flour, baking soda and salt; set aside.

4.   In a medium bowl, cream together the cannabis butter, normal butter, brown sugar and white sugar until well blended. Beat in the vanilla, egg and egg yolk until light and creamy.

5.   Mix in the sifted ingredients until just blended. Stir in the chocolate chips by hand using a wooden spoon.

6.   Drop cookie dough 1/4 cup at a time onto the prepared cookie sheets. Cookies should be about 3 inches apart.

7.   Bake for 15 to 17 minutes in the preheated oven, or until the edges are lightly toasted. Cool on baking sheets for a few minutes before transferring to wire racks to cool completely.

28. No-Bake Cannabis Cookie

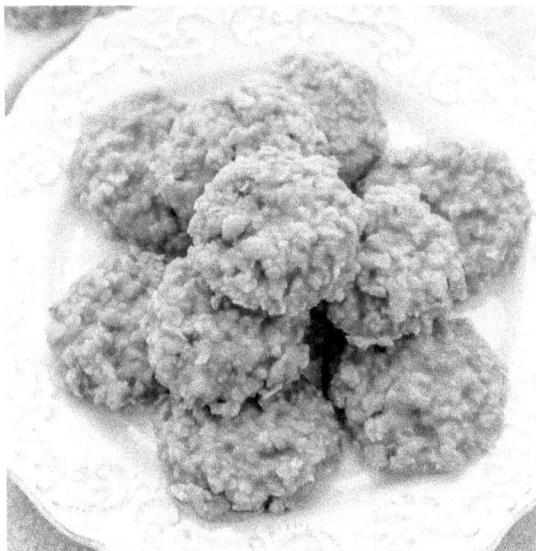

Ingredients:

1/2 cup melted cannabis butter

1 ½ cups Graham cracker crumbs

One pound confectioners' sugar (3 to 3 1/2 cups) 1 ½ CUPS peanut butter

1/2 cup butter, melted

1 (12 ounces) bag milk chocolate chips

Directions:

1.   Combine Graham cracker crumbs, sugar and peanut butter; mix well.

2.   Blend in the melted cannabis butter until well combined.

3.   Press mixture evenly into a 9 x 13-inch pan.

4.   Melt chocolate chips in microwave or in a double boiler.

5.   Spread over peanut butter mixture.

6.   Chill until just set and cut into bars. (These are very hard to cut if the chocolate gets "rock hard".)

29. Chocolate Bananas

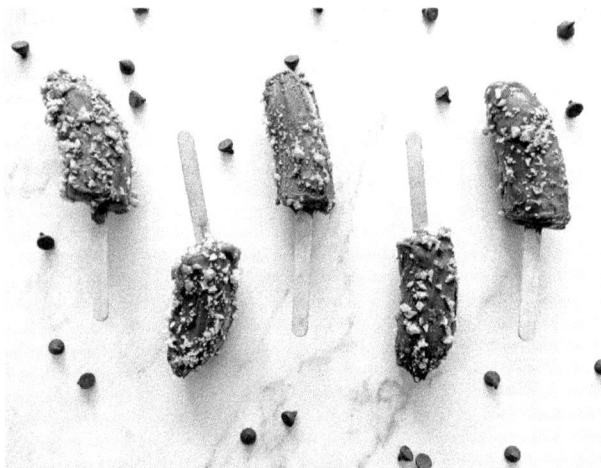

Easy recipe for cannabis-infused chocolate-dipped bananas.

Ingredients:

½ cup cannabutter

3 ripe but firm bananas

1 pound dark chocolate, chopped, or semisweet chocolate chips

1/2 cup granola, chopped pecans and walnuts, or sprinkles (optional)

Directions:

1.   Line a baking sheet with nonstick foil or parchment paper.

2.   Cut the bananas in half and insert a popsicle stick into each half, as shown.

3.   Place them on the baking sheet and freeze for 15 minutes.

4.   Melt the cannabutter over a low heat and then set it aside.

5.   Melt chocolate in the same double boiler until smooth. Add the cannabutter to the chocolate as it's melting. Gently mix the cannabutter into the chocolate.

6.   Roll each banana half in the chocolate, then quickly sprinkle with your topping (if using).

7.   Freeze until the chocolate sets, 30 minutes.

8.   Serve and then enjoy! Or freeze in an airtight container for up to a week.

30.Creamy Stuffed Cannabis-Infused Pancakes

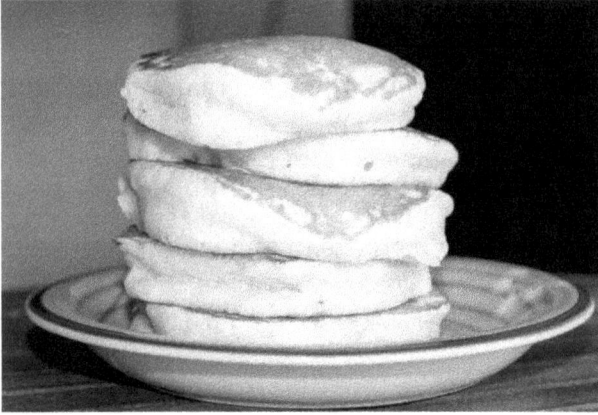

Ingredients:

1   cup cannabis milk 1 egg

2   tablespoons vegetable oil 1 teaspoon salt

2 tablespoons sugar

1   cup flour

2   teaspoons baking powder (for the filling) 1 cup cream cheese

Chopped strawberries Blueberries

2 tablespoons vanilla sugar 1/2 cup whipping cream

Directions:

1.   In a large bowl, sift together the flour, baking powder, salt, and sugar. Make a well in the center and pour in the milk, egg and vegetable oil; mix until smooth.

2.   Heat a lightly oiled griddle or frying pan over medium-high to low heat. Pour or scoop the batter onto the griddle. Brown on both sides and serve hot.

For Filling:

1.   In a medium mixing bowl, beat the softened cream cheese until smooth.

2.   Add whipping cream and vanilla. Beat mixture until combined. Stir in both berries and sugar.

3.   To serve, spoon 2/3 tablespoons of filling onto each thin pancake.

4.   Serve with chocolate sauce.

31. Chocolate Weed Brownies

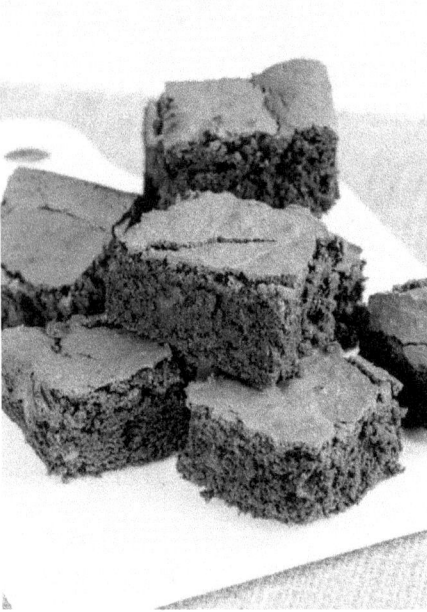

Ingredients:

1/4 cup cannabis butter 1/4 cup normal butter 2 eggs

1 teaspoon vanilla extract

1/3 cup unsweetened cocoa powder 1/2 cup all-purpose flour

1/4 teaspoon salt

1/4 teaspoon baking powder

For the Frosting:

3 tablespoons butter, softened

1 teaspoon cannabis butter, softened 1 tablespoon honey

1 teaspoon vanilla extract 1 cup confectioners' sugar

Directions:

1. Preheat oven to 330 degrees F.

2. Grease and flour an 8-inch square pan.

3. In a large saucepan, on very low heat, melt 1/4 cup butter and 1/4 cup cannabis butter. Remove from heat, and stir in sugar, eggs and 1 teaspoon

vanilla. Beat in 1/3 cup cocoa, 1/2 cup flour, salt and baking powder. Spread batter into prepared pan.

4. Bake in preheated oven for 25 to 30 minutes. Do not overcook.

For Frosting:

1. Combine 3 tablespoons softened butter and 1 teaspoon cannabis butter; add 3 tablespoons cocoa, honey, 1 teaspoon vanilla extract, and 1 cup confectioners' sugar. Stir until smooth.

2. Frost brownies while they are still warm.

32. Cannabis Chocolate Birthday Cake

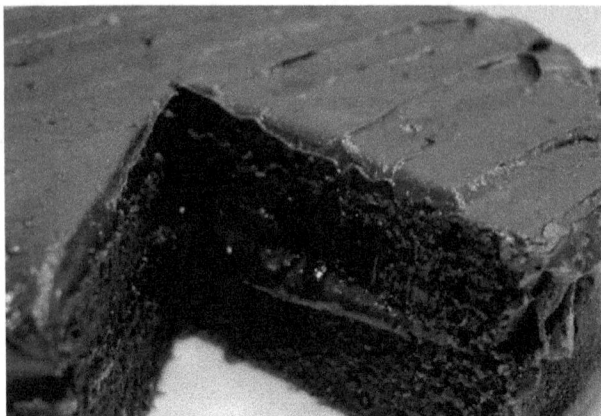

Ingredients:

1/2 cup of cannabis butter

8 heaping tablespoons cocoa, plus more for dusting 4 cups all-purpose flour

4 cups sugar

1/2 teaspoon salt

2 cups boiling water 1 cup buttermilk

2 teaspoons baking soda

2   teaspoons vanilla extract 4 whole eggs, beaten

For Frosting:

3   cups heavy cream

24 ounces semisweet chocolate, broken into pieces 2 teaspoons vanilla extract

Directions:

For Cake:

1.   Preheat the oven to 350 degrees F. Heavily grease and dust four 9-inch round cake pans with cocoa.

2.   In a mixing bowl, combine the flour, sugar and salt.

3.   In a saucepan, melt the cannabis butter on very low heat. Add the cocoa. Stir together. Add the boiling water; allow the mixture to simmer on low for 30 seconds, and then turn off the heat. Pour over the flour mixture and stir lightly to cool.

4.   Combine the buttermilk, baking soda, vanilla and beaten eggs. Stir the buttermilk mixture into the butter/chocolate mixture.

5.   Divide the batter among the prepared cake pans and bake for 20 minutes.

6.   Cool completely before icing. Refrigerate the layers after cooling for best results.

For Frosting:

1.   Heat the cream until very hot, and then pour over the chocolate pieces. Stir to completely melt, and then pour into the bowl of an electric mixer. Refrigerate to cool.

2.   Once completely cooled, add the vanilla and beat with an electric mixer until light and airy.

3.   Frost the cake in between each layer, on the top and around the sides.

33. Cannabis Banana Muffins

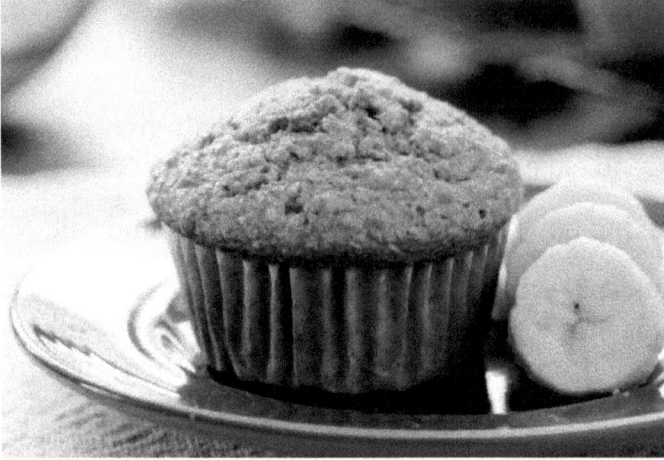

Ingredients:

1/4 cup cannabis oil

2 1/2 cups unbleached all-purpose flour 1/2 teaspoon baking soda

3/4 cup dark brown sugar

1/4 teaspoon ground cinnamon

2 cups smashed bananas (about 4 to 6 bananas) 1/2 cup milk

2 large eggs, at room temperature 1/8 teaspoon fine salt

1/2 teaspoon pure vanilla extract 3/4 cups chopped walnuts

Directions:

1.   Preheat the oven to 350 degrees F. Lightly brush a 12-muffin tin with butter and set aside.

2.   Whisk the flour, baking soda, brown sugar and cinnamon together in a medium bowl, set aside.

3.   Whisk the banana, cannabis oil, milk, eggs, salt and vanilla in a large measuring cup with a spout or another bowl.

4.   Make a small well in the center of the dry ingredients. Pour wet ingredients into the center; then stir with a wooden spoon until the dry ingredients are moistened but still lumpy. Do not overmix the batter or your

muffins will become dense. Gently stir in the nuts. Divide the batter evenly into the muffin tin.

5.   Bake until golden brown, about 25 minutes, rotating the pan halfway through the cooking. (Insert a toothpick into the center of a muffin to check if it is done. Toothpick should come out clean.)

6.   Cool muffins in the pan on a rack for a couple minutes. Turn the muffins out of the pan and cool on the rack. Serve warm or at room temperature.

34. Cannabis Coconut Creme Brûlée

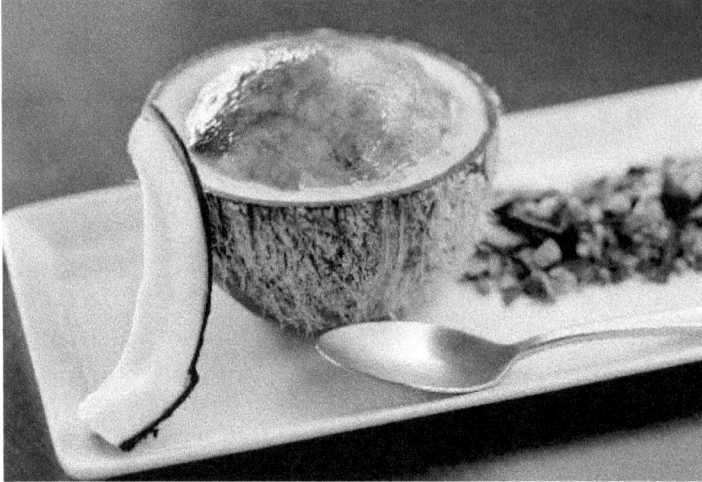

Ingredients:

2 tablespoons cannabis coconut oil 1 cup unsweetened coconut milk

1 cup heavy cream

1 teaspoon imitation coconut extract 4 large eggs

8 to 9 tablespoons sugar

Directions:

1.   Preheat the oven to 325 degrees F.

2.   Combine the coconut milk, cream and coconut extract in a small saucepan over medium-high heat and bring to a boil. Once at a boil, remove from the heat. Add coconut oil

3.   Meanwhile, whisk together the eggs and 5 tablespoons sugar in a bowl until combined.

4.   Slowly whisk the heated cream mixture into the eggs, stirring constantly.

5.   Divide the mixture among six, heat-safe 5-ounce coffee mugs or oven- safe ramekins, filling them about 3/4 of the way up. Put them in a baking dish, and add enough warm water to the baking dish so that it comes halfway up the sides of the coffee mugs.

6.   Bake until the center is nearly set. Baking time will depend on the height of your coffee mug or ramekin. Bake time is 10 minutes for every 1/2 inch of height. For a 1-inch vessel, bake the creme brulees about 20 minutes. For a 2-inch vessel, bake the creme brulees about 40 minutes.

7.   Remove from the oven and allow to completely cool in the water bath, then refrigerate 15 to 20 minutes before serving.

8.   Before serving, sprinkle the tops with a heavy layer of sugar. Use a hand torch or heat under the broiler for 2 to 3 minutes.

35. Cannabis Tiramisu

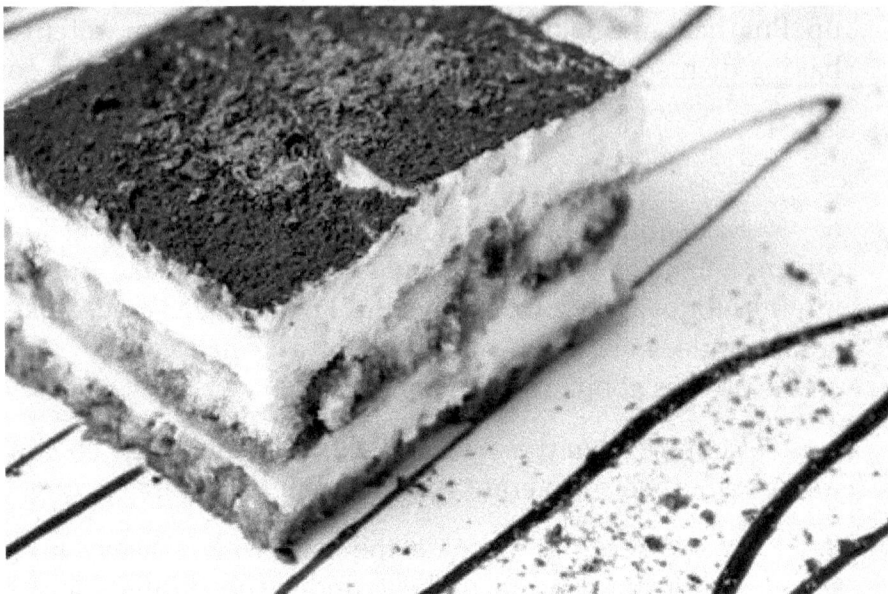

Ingredients:

6 extra-large egg yolks, at room temperature 1/4 cup sugar

1/2 cup good dark rum, divided

1 1/2 cups brewed espresso, divided 3 tablespoons cannabis coconut oil 16 to 17 ounces mascarpone cheese 30 Italian ladyfingers or savoiardi

Bittersweet chocolate, shaved or grated Confectioners' sugar (optional)

Directions:

1.   Whisk the egg yolks and sugar in the bowl of an electric mixer fitted with the whisk attachment on high speed for about 5 minutes, or until very thick and light yellow. Lower the speed to medium and add 1/4 cup rum, 1/4 cup espresso, 2 tablespoons cannabis coconut oil and the mascarpone. Whisk until smooth.

2.   Combine the remaining 1/4 cup rum and 1 1/4 cups espresso with 1 tablespoon cannabis coconut oil in a shallow bowl. Dip 1 side of each ladyfinger in the espresso/rum mixture and line the bottom of a 9x12x2- inch dish. Pour half the espresso cream mixture evenly on top. Dip 1 side of the remaining ladyfingers in the espresso/rum mixture and place them in a

second layer in the dish. Pour the rest of the espresso cream over the top. Smooth the top and cover with plastic wrap. Refrigerate overnight.

3.   Before serving, sprinkle the top with shaved chocolate and dust lightly with confectioners' sugar, if desired.

36. Chocolate Ganache Cannabis Cupcakes

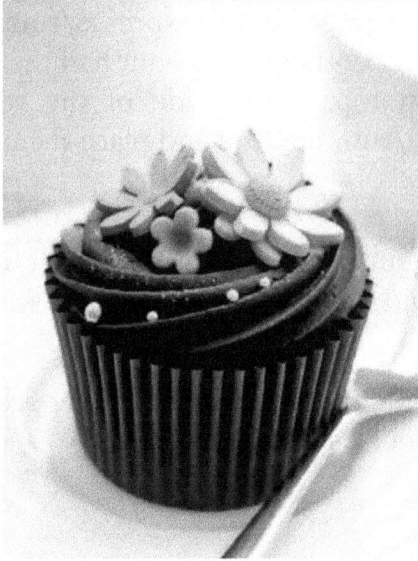

Ingredients:

1/4 cup cannabis butter 1 cup sugar

4 extra-large eggs, at room temperature

16 fluid ounces Hershey's chocolate syrup 1 tablespoon pure vanilla extract

1 cup all-purpose flour

1 teaspoon instant coffee granules

For Ganache:

1/2 cup heavy cream

8 ounces good-quality, semisweet chocolate chips 1/2 teaspoon instant coffee granules

Directions:

1.   Preheat the oven to 325 degrees F. Line a muffin pan with paper liners.

2.   Cream the cannabis butter and sugar in the bowl of an electric mixer fitted with the paddle attachment until light and fluffy. Add the eggs, 1 at a time. Mix in the chocolate syrup and vanilla. Add the flour and coffee granules and mix until just combined. Don't overbeat or the cupcakes will be tough.

3.   Scoop the batter into the muffin cups and bake for 30 minutes, or until just set in the middle. Don't overbake! Let cool thoroughly in the muffin pan.

For Ganache:

1.   Cook the heavy cream, chocolate chips and instant coffee in the top of a double boiler over simmering water until smooth and warm, stirring occasionally.

2.   Dip the tops of the cupcakes into the ganache. Do not refrigerate.

37. Cannabis Thumbprint Tea Cookies Recipe

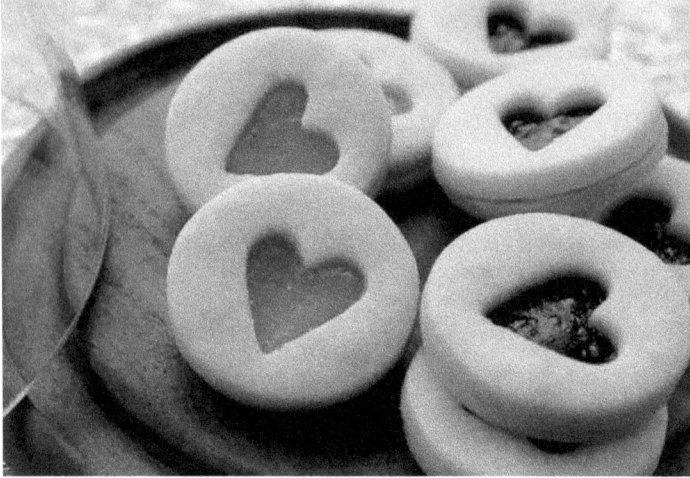

Yield: 3 Dozen Thumbprint Tea Cookies

Whether they're for a crowd or just you, these thumbprint cookies are sure to dazzle and delight in both flavor and effect. Don't forget to label the cookie jar.

Ingredients:

1 cup (4:20) butter and cannabutter 1/3 cup powdered sugar

1 teaspoon vanilla 1 & 2/3 cups flour

Fruit Filling:

8 oz. jar (your choice) of favorite jam/preserve/jelly, 4:20 vg tincture

Chocolate Filling:

12 oz. (your choice) of chocolate, cannabis oil

Directions:

1.   Pre-heat oven to 350 F.

2.   In a large mixing bowl, cream together cannabis butter and powdered sugar until light and fluffy. Fold in vanilla.

3.   Mix in flour and place finished dough into refrigerator for 30 min.

4.   Line cookie trays with parchment paper. Form dough into 1" balls, then place onto tray, 12 to a tray. Once the cookies have cooled, use the back of a spoon to make indentations into the cookies that will be filled later. Cook for 8-10 minutes or until golden brown. Let cool completely before filling.

For Fruit Filling:

1.   Using your favorite jam/jelly/preserve, place contents of one jar into a medium saucepot on low heat. Add 2 tablespoons of water and heat until warm and manageable, then remove from heat. Stir in 2-3 tablespoons of 4:20 VG Tincture (can be adjusted to your personal levels). Fill each cookie and let sit for 15 minutes before placing in refrigerator for 30 minutes.

For Chocolate Filling:

1. Melt your chocolate of choice 1-2 minutes in microwave, then stir in 2- 3 tablespoons 4:20 oil (can be adjusted to your personal levels). Fill each cookie and let sit for 15 minutes before placing into refrigerator for 30 minutes.

38. No-Bake Fudge

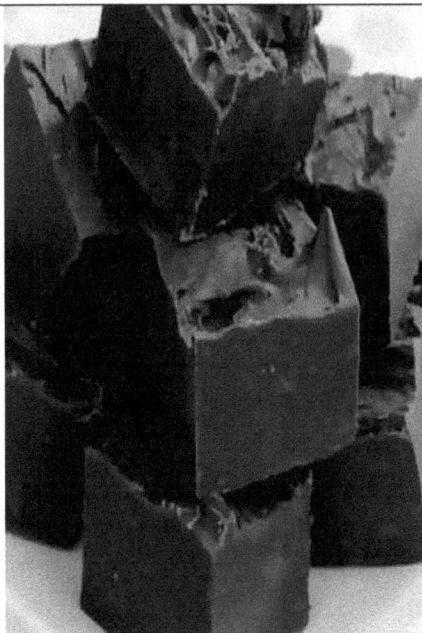

This delicious cannabis-infused fudge requires no baking. Be warned – it's potent stuff!

Ingredients:

7 cups (2 lbs) powdered sugar 1 cup of Hershey's cocoa

1 lb (4 sticks) of cannabutter 1 teaspoon of vanilla essence 1 cup of peanut butter

Directions:

1.   Melt the butter and peanut butter in a saucepan or double boiler, and add the vanilla essence

2.   In a large bowl, mix together the powdered sugar and cocoa.

3.   Add the melted ingredients and mix well

4.   Press into a flat pan, and place in the fridge until firm

39. Chocolate-Dipped Weed Cherries

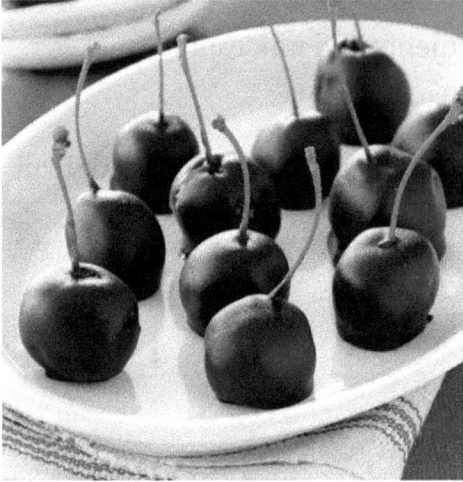

Time Required: 2 hours 15 minutes Yield: 24 Chocolate Cannabis Cherries

Ingredients:

1 cup dark chocolate chips 1 cup milk chocolate chips

¼ cup cannabis coconut oil

24 cherries with stems (washed and dried; if you use fresh cherries, remember to remove the pit!)

Directions:

1.   Heat milk chocolate chips, dark chocolate chips and cannabis coconut oil in a microwave safe bowl. Remove and stir every 20 seconds until melted.

Chocolate should be warm but not hot.

2.   Dip dry cherries by the stems in chocolate, one at a time, allowing excess chocolate to drip back into bowl.

3.   Set cherries on a wax paper-lined plate to dry. Repeat until all cherries are coated. Save extra chocolate on the side. (You will dip the cherries again.)

4.   Chill cherries in the refrigerator for 1 hour.

5.   Warm the chocolate sauce back up and remove cherries from the refrigerator.

6.   Dip each cherry in the chocolate sauce for a second time. Return cherries to the refrigerator to chill for 1 hour before serving.

7.   Store extra cherries in the refrigerator.

40. Cannabutter Pound Cake

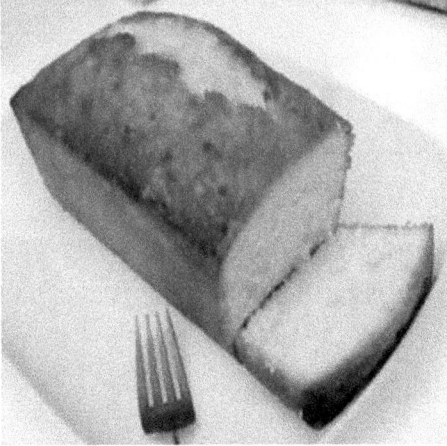

Prep Time: 10 minutes Cook Time: 80 minutes

This classic cake is elevated with the addition of cream cheese!

Ingredients:

½ cup cannabutter, softened 1 cup real butter, softened

1 (8 oz) package cream cheese, softened 3 cups white sugar

6 eggs

3 cups all-purpose flour 1 teaspoon vanilla extract

Directions:

1.   Heat oven to 325 degrees F. Spray a 9×5 bread pan with nonstick spray.

2.   With an electric mixer, mix everything except the flour until combined. Once combined, add flour. Mix until combined.

3.   Pour mixture into 9×5 pan. Bake 80 minutes.

4.   Let it cool !

41. Cannabis Taffy

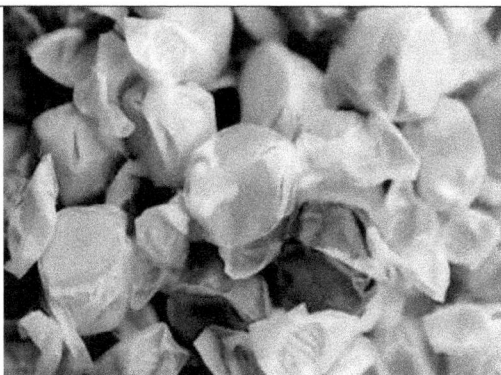

Prep TIme: 45 minutes Yield: 3 to 4 dozen pieces

Ingredients:

1½ mugs cocoa sugar

½ glass cannabis corn syrup

3 tablespoons cannabutter (or customary margarine) 1½ teaspoons salt

1½ teaspoons vanilla extract

Directions:

1.   Join cocoa sugar, corn syrup, cannabutter and water in a pan. Heat, mixing infrequently, until temperature comes to 256 degrees F.

2.   Include salt and cannabis corn syrup to pot and blend.

3.   Pour blend onto a lubed marble/stone section, and permit to cool until you can securely touch it.

4.   Stretch out taffy until it is light in shading, including vanilla extract as you extend.

5.   Haul out strings of taffy that are 1 inch in measurement. Oil scissors and softly cut taffy into chomp size pieces.

6.   Wrap every individual bit of taffy in wax paper. Twist ends to close.

42. Cannabis Corn Syrup

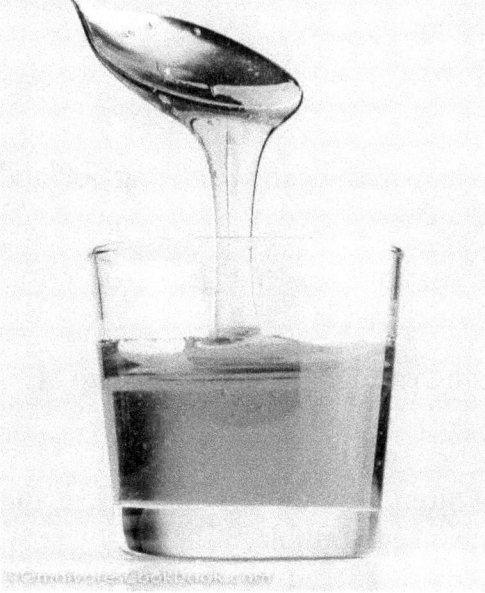

There are an assortment of cannabis corn syrup formulas that call for anywhere from ¼ ounce to 4 ounces of cannabis for each 6 measures of corn syrup. The power of the formulas on this site relies upon the centralization of cannabis in your key fixing. The measure of cannabis in the formula beneath is only a proposal and can be altered by individual dose.

Time Required: 4 hours (suggested minimum)

Ingredients:

Vast pot or slow cooker 3 glasses light corn syrup

1   ounce finely ground cannabis Cheesecloth

Spoon

Tupperware holder with cover

Elastic band (one that will extend around the edge of your Tupperware)

Directions:

1. Pour the light corn syrup in the pan or stewing pot, and set on low/medium warmth.

2. Let the syrup warm up until it is hot; however, ensure it doesn't bubble.

3. Add your finely ground cannabis to the hot syrup.

4. Blend the cannabis often as it douses for no less than 4 hours. Try not to give it a chance to bubble.

5. Set up your Tupperware holder by taking 2 sheets of the cheesecloth and securing it over the cover of the dish utilizing the elastic band. Turn heat off and let blend cool down somewhat.

6. Pour the cannabis corn syrup blend gradually over the highest point of the cheesecloth and into the holder. Rehash this progression as important to strain the greater part of the plant from the syrup.

7. Permit syrup to cool. Store the cannabis corn syrup in an impenetrable holder and keep it in a cool, dim spot.

43. Weed Candy

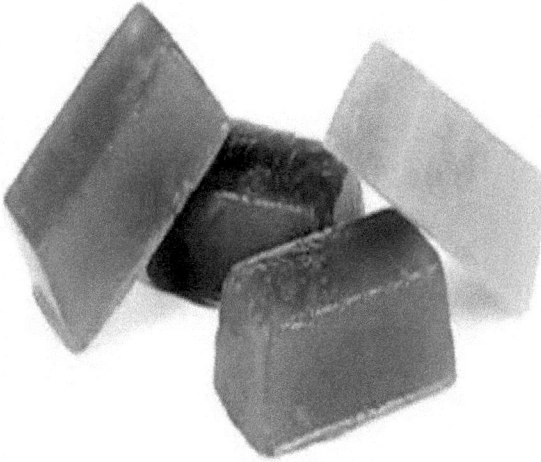

Time Required: 25 minutes Yield: 3 to 4 dozen pieces

Ingredients:

2   cups sugar

1¼ cup cannabis corn syrup 1 cup water

Food coloring/flavoring of your choice

Directions:

1.   Heat sugar, cannabis corn syrup and water in saucepan over medium heat.

2.   Stir until all sugars are dissolved. Bring to a 300 degree boil.

3.   Add food coloring and flavoring slowly. Stir well.

4.   Turn off heat. Carefully and quickly pour liquid into candy molds before it hardens.

5.   Remove candy from mold once it is finished cooling. Toss candy in sugar, if desired.

44. Cannabis Caramel Candy

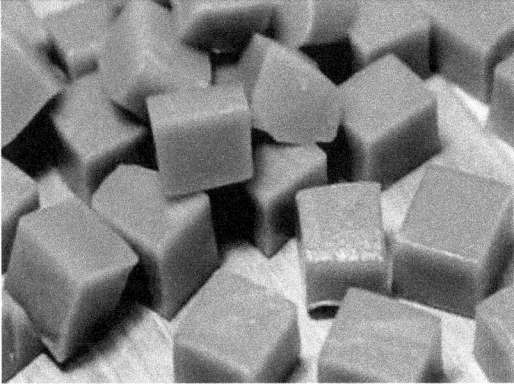

Time Required: 25 minutes Yield: 3 to 4 dozen pieces

Ingredients:

1   cup cannabutter

2   ¼ cups brown sugar Dash salt

1 cup light corn syrup

14 ounces sweetened condensed milk (canned) 1 teaspoon vanilla

Extract

Directions:

1.   Melt cannabutter slowly in saucepan.

2.   Stir in brown sugar and salt until combined.

3.   Stir in light corn syrup.

4.   Add milk slowly while constantly stirring.

5.   Cook mixture over medium heat until candy begins to get firmer (usually 12 to 15 minutes).

6.   Remove saucepan from heat and stir in the vanilla extract.

7.   Pour mixture into 9x13 pan. Allow candy to cool down.

8.   Cut, serve and store.

45. Caramel Cashew Squares

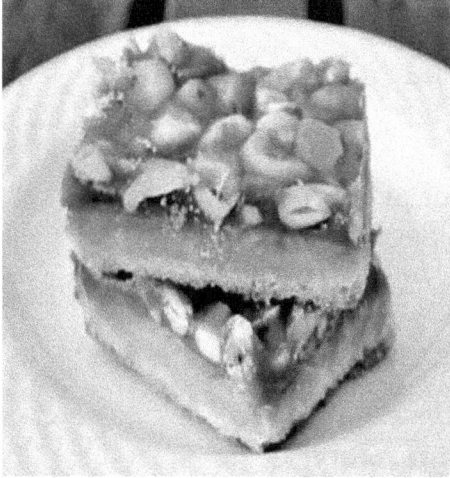

This recipe is topped with salted cashews and gooey caramel. It is rich, sweet and includes cannabutter! Cannabis Caramel Cashew Squares are an effortless dessert and irresistibly delicious.

Ingredients:

For Crust:

1/3 cup firmly packed brown sugar

4 tablespoons butter (2 cannabutter, 2 regular) 1 cup all-purpose flour

1/4 teaspoon salt

For Topping:

1/2 cup butterscotch-flavored baking chips 1/4 cup light corn syrup

2 tablespoons cannabutter

1 cup chopped salted cashews

Directions:

1. Heat oven to 350°F.

2. Place brown sugar in medium bowl.

3. Add 4 tablespoons of butter, and mix with brown sugar in a blender until it resembles coarse crumbs.

4. Add flour and salt. Mix well.

5. Press mixture onto bottom of the ungreased 8-inch square baking pan.

6. Bake for 11-13 minutes and let set.

7. Melt butterscotch chips, corn syrup and 2 tablespoons cannabutter in 2- quart saucepan over low heat, stirring occasionally.

8. Remove from heat. Stir in cashews.

9. Pour cashew mixture over the crust.

10. Continue baking for 8-10 minutes or until it starts to bubble.

11. Set and cool completely.

12. Cover; store refrigerated. Cut into bars.

46. Dank Cheesecake

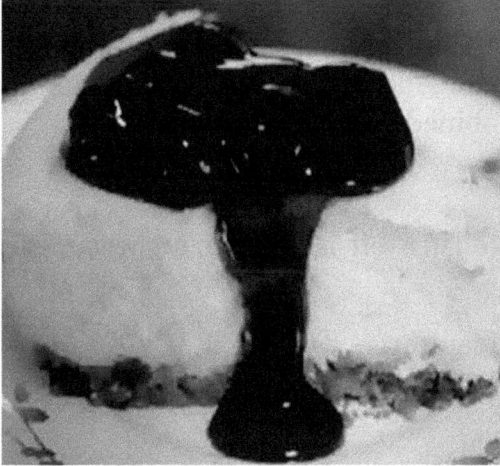

Try topping your Dank Cheesecake with fruit and other sweets!

Ingredients:

1/3 cup cannabutter, softened

1   (9 oz) premade Graham cracker crust

2   (8 oz) packages cream cheese, softened

¾ cup white sugar 1/3 cup milk

2 eggs

½ cup sour cream

1   ½ teaspoons vanilla extract

2   tablespoons all-purpose flour

Directions:

1.	Heat oven to 350 degrees F. Remove plastic from premade crust.

2.	With an electric mixer, mix cannabutter, cream cheese and sugar until combined. Add milk, eggs, sour cream, vanilla and flour. Mix until combined. Pour mixture into crust.

3.	Bake 1 hour. Turn off heat. Leave cheesecake in closed oven for 5 hours.

4.	Store in refrigerator.

47. Flourless Canna Chocolate Cake

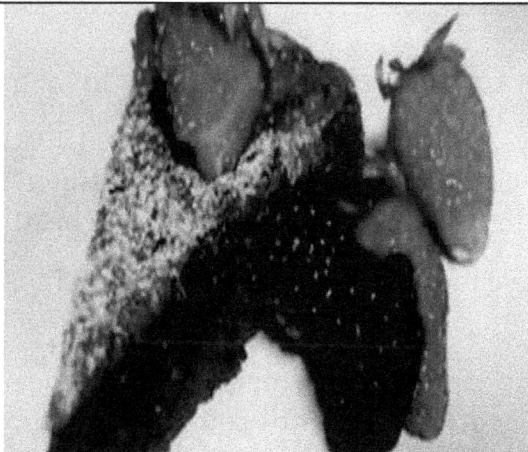

Time Required: 9 hours Prep Time: 20 minutes Cook Time: 45 minutes

Whether or not you're sensitive to gluten, this cake is still awesome!

Ingredients:

½ cup cannabutter, melted

½ cup real butter, melted

½ cup water

¼ tsp salt

¾ cup white sugar

18 (1 oz) pieces bittersweet Baker's chocolate 6 eggs

Directions:

1.   Heat oven to 300 degrees F. Spray a 10" pie dish with nonstick spray.

2.   In a saucepan and on medium heat, stir water, sugar and salt until everything has dissolved. Remove from heat.

3.   Microwave chocolate until melted. Be careful not to burn it.

4.   With an electric mixer, mix melted chocolate, cannabutter, real butter and sugar mixture until combined. Mix in the eggs, two at a time until combined.

5.   Pour mixture into pie dish. Set pie dish in a larger pan, and fill the larger pan with water until the water is ½ way to the top of the pie dish.

6.   Bake 45 minutes.

7.   Refrigerate 8 hours.

48. Chronic Carrot Cake

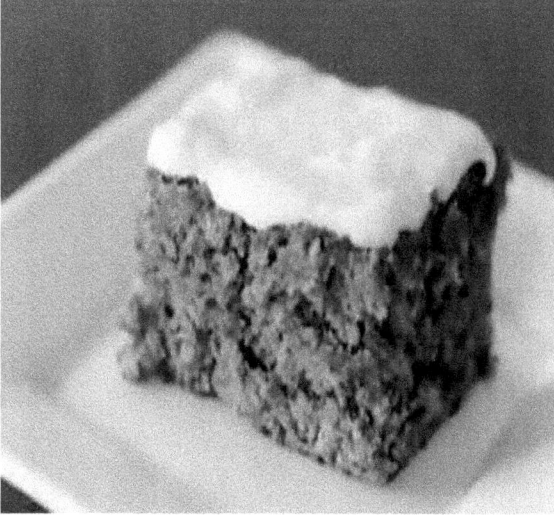

This cannabis-infused carrot cake is a healthy and fun dessert!

Ingredients:

For Cake:

2   cups all-purpose flour 1 teaspoon baking soda

2   teaspoons ground cinnamon 1/4 teaspoon salt

3   eggs

3/4 cup buttermilk 1 cup cannaoil

1   1/2 cups sugar

2   teaspoons vanilla extract 2 1/2 cups shredded carrots 1 cup flaked coconut

1 cup chopped walnuts 1 cup raisins

For Frosting:

1/2 cup butter, softened (or cannabutter)

1 cup cream cheese (or canna cream cheese) 4 cups powdered sugar

1   teaspoon vanilla extract

Directions:

1.   Preheat oven to 350 degrees F.

2.   Sift together flour, baking soda, salt and cinnamon in a medium-sized bowl. Set aside.

3.   Combine eggs, buttermilk, cannaoil, sugar and vanilla in a separate bowl, mix well.

4.   Add flour mixture to the cannaoil mixture, stir well.

5.   Combine shredded carrots, coconut, walnuts and raisins in a separate bowl.

6.   Add carrot mixture to batter and mix thoroughly.

7.   Pour batter into a greased cake pan and bake for 1 hour or until toothpick comes out clean.

8.   Remove cake from oven and let cool.

9.   Mix cream cheese, butter, milk and vanilla together while cake is cooling.

10.   Frost cake with icing. Store in refrigerator.

11.   In a medium bowl, combine butter, cream cheese, powdered sugar and vanilla extract to make the frosting. Beat until the mixture is smooth and creamy.

12.   Frost the cooled cake. Cut and serve.

49. Pumpkin Roll-It-Up Cake

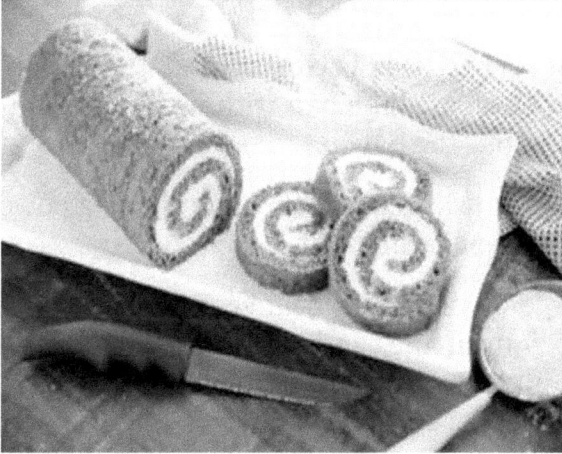

Time Required: 1 hour 40 minutes Serves: 8

Ingredients:

Cake:

1/4 cup confectioner's sugar for dusting towel 3/4 cup all-purpose flour

1/2 teaspoon baking powder 1/2 teaspoon baking soda

2   teaspoons pumpkin pie spice 1/4 teaspoon salt

3   large eggs

1 cup granulated sugar 2/3 cup canned pumpkin

For Filling:

1 package cream cheese, softened, 8 ounces

3 tablespoons cannabis-infused butter, softened 5 tablespoons butter, softened

1 teaspoon vanilla extract 1 1/4 cups powdered sugar

Directions:

For Cake:

1.   Preheat oven to 375° F. Grease a 12x17 inch jellyroll pan or cookie sheet with sides. Line pan with wax or parchment paper, and grease and flour the paper.

2.   In a small bowl, combine the flour, baking powder, baking soda, pumpkin pie spice and salt.

3.   In a large mixing bowl, beat eggs and sugar together with an electric mixer until thick and pale yellow, about 2 minutes. Stir in canned pumpkin until well combined. Stir in flour mixture just until combined.

4.   Pour mixture into prepared pan.

5.   Use a rubber spatula to smooth the batter out to the edges in an even layer, and bake 12 - 15 minutes or until cake springs back when touched.

6.   While cake is baking, prepare clean kitchen towel by laying on the counter and dusting evenly with the powdered sugar.

7.   When cake is done, immediately invert onto kitchen towel.

8.   Peel off the parchment paper.

9.   Starting at the shorter end of the towel, gently and loosely roll the cake inside of the towel. (The towel will be wrapped up inside the cake roll.) Move to a rack and cool completely before filling.

For Filling:

1.   Combine all ingredients in a medium size bowl and beat until fluffy.

2.   When cake is cool, unroll from towel and spread the cream cheese filling over the cake up to the edges.

3.   Re-roll cake and wrap in plastic wrap. Refrigerate for at least 1 hour.

4.   Dust with powdered sugar just before serving and slice crosswise into pieces.

50. Pumpkin Pot Brownies

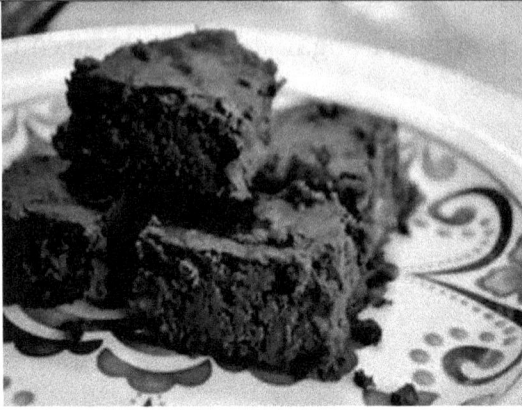

Ingredients:

2/3 cup packed brown sugar 1/2 cup canned pumpkin

1   whole egg

2   egg whites

1/4 cup cannabutter

1 cup all-purpose flour

1 teaspoon baking powder

1   teaspoon unsweetened cocoa powder 1/2 teaspoon ground cinnamon

1/2 teaspoon ground allspice 1/4 teaspoon salt

1/4 teaspoon ground nutmeg

1/3 cup miniature semisweet chocolate pieces

Directions:

1.   Preheat oven to 350 degrees F.

2.   In a large mixing bowl, combine brown sugar, pumpkin, the whole egg, egg whites and oil.

3.   Beat with an electric mixer on medium speed until blended.

4.   Add flour, baking powder, cocoa powder, cinnamon, allspice, salt and nutmeg.

5.   Beat on low speed until smooth. Stir in semisweet chocolate pieces.

6.   Spray an 11×7 inch baking pan with nonstick coating.

7.   Pour batter into pan. Spread evenly.

8.   Bake 15 to 20 minutes or until a toothpick inserted near the center comes out clean.

51. Rocky Road Marijuana Brownies

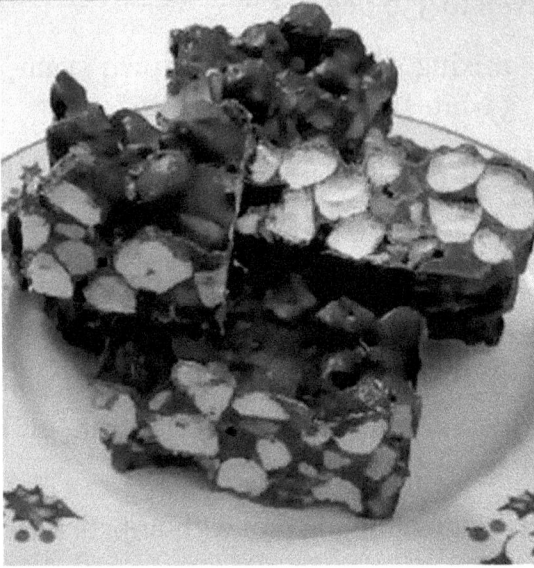

Yield: 12 brownies

Ingredients:

1/2 cup cannabis-infused butter 1/8 cup butter

2   ounces unsweetened chocolate

4 ounces bittersweet or semisweet chocolate 3/4 cup all-purpose flour

1/2 teaspoon salt

1 cup granulated sugar 2 large eggs

1 teaspoon vanilla extract

3/4 cup toasted almond slices 1 cup miniature marshmallows

Directions:

1.   Preheat the oven to 350 degrees F. Line an 8-inch square baking pan with aluminum foil, and grease foil with either butter or vegetable shortening.

2.   marijuana brownies, lining the pan

3.   Melt the cannabutter, butter and chocolates over low heat in a medium saucepan stirring frequently. Set aside to cool for 5 minutes.

4.   Stir together the flour and salt; set aside.

5.   Stir the sugar into the melted cannabutter until well combined.

6.   Beat in the eggs and vanilla and continue mixing until well incorporated.

7.   Mix in the flour and salt until just incorporated.

8.   Reserve 1/2 cup of the brownie batter, and spread the remainder into the prepared pan.

9.   Bake batter in the pan for about 20 minutes. While it is baking, prepare the topping by stirring together the reserved batter with the toasted almonds and marshmallows.

10.   After batter in pan has baked for 20 minute, remove from oven.

11.   Spread topping over par-baked brownies and return to oven. Bake for about 10 more minutes or until marshmallows are browned and a toothpick inserted in the center comes out with just a few moist crumbs clinging to it.

12.   Let cool in pan before using the foil to lift out the brownies and slice.

52. Microwave Peanut Butter Swirl Brownie

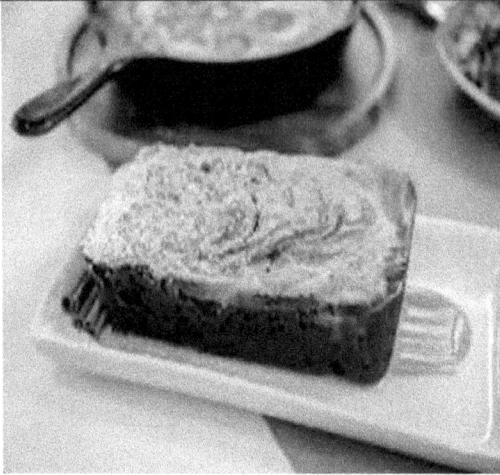

Ingredients:

2   tablespoons cannabutter, softened 2 tablespoons sugar

1 1/2 tablespoons brown sugar 1 tablespoon cocoa powder

1 egg yolk

3 tablespoons flour Pinch of salt Splash of vanilla

1 tablespoon creamy peanut butter

Directions:

1.   Mix the cannabutter, sugar, brown sugar, vanilla and egg yolk until smooth.

2.   Stir in the salt and flour until well combined. Stir chocolate chips in last.

3.   Pour into a ramekin or mug, then dot the top with peanut butter.

4.   Swirl lightly with a butter knife.

5.   Microwave for 45-75 seconds in the microwave until just done.

53. CannaCrack

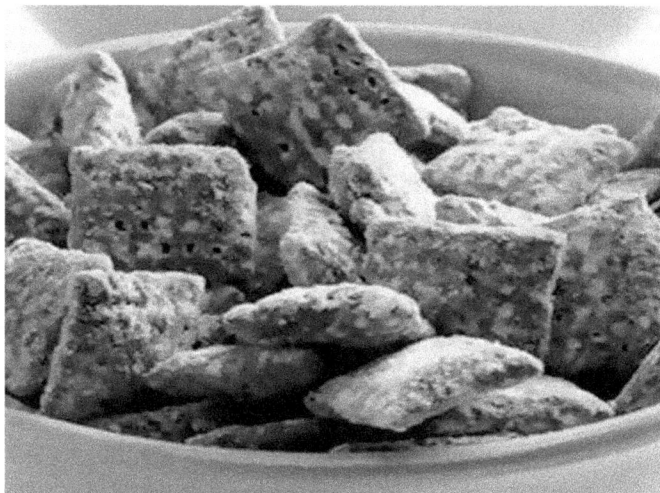

Prep Time: 5 minutes Cook Time: 15 minutes

CannaCrack is so good that you may need to check in to rehab!

Ingredients:

1/3 cup cannabutter 9 cups Chex cereal

1 cup semisweet chocolate chips

½ cup peanut butter

1 teaspoon vanilla extract 1 ½ cups powdered sugar

Directions:

1.   Place the cereal into a 1 gallon Ziplock freezer bag.

2.   In a saucepan and on medium heat, add everything except the powdered sugar. Stir until melted and combined.

3.   Pour the chocolate mixture onto the cereal inside the Ziplock bag. Seal the bag and shake it until all the cereal is coated with the chocolate mixture. Once the cereal is coated, pour the powdered sugar into the Ziplock bag, seal it, and shake it until the powdered sugar has coated everything.

4.   Let cool, store in the same Ziplock bag, and eat with caution.

54. Oven-Baked Donut Holes

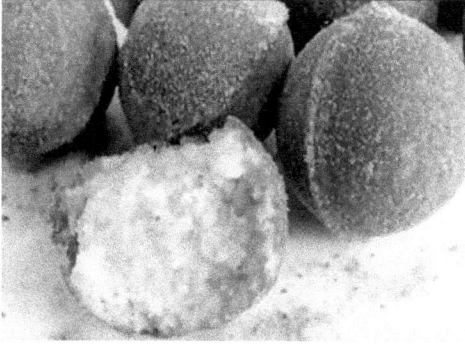

Time Required: 50 minutes

These donuts can be filled with your favorite pudding, jelly or sweet cream.

Ingredients:

1 cup white sugar

½ cup cannabutter, melted

¾ teaspoon ground nutmeg

½ cup milk

1 teaspoon baking powder 1 cup all purpose flour

1 teaspoon ground cinnamon

Directions:

1.   Heat oven to 350 degrees F. Spray all of the cups of a mini-muffin pan with nonstick cooking spray.

2.   With an electric stand mixer, mix ½ cup sugar, nutmeg, ¼ cup cannabutter, milk, baking powder and flour until combined

3.   Fill mini-muffin cups ½ way full with donut mix. Bake 20 minutes.

4.   When donuts are in oven, take 2 separate bowls and put ¼ cup melted cannabutter in one, and ½ cup sugar with cinnamon in the other.

5.   When donuts have finished baking, remove them from the mini-muffin pan and, one-at-a-time, dip them first in the melted cannabutter followed by coating them with the cinnamon sugar.

6.   Let cool.

55. Peanut Butter Bud Bars

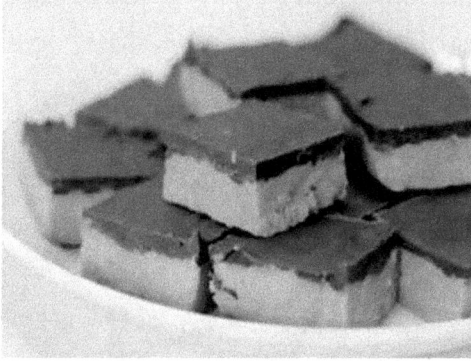

Peanut Butter Bud Bars are a fast snack to make and are a great way to relax at the end of the day!

Ingredients:

½ cup cannabutter, melted

½ cup regular butter, melted

1 tablespoon decarb seasoning 2 cups Graham cracker crumbs 2 cups powdered sugar

1 cup + 4 tablespoons creamy peanut butter 1 ½ cups semisweet chocolate chips

Directions:

1.   In a bowl, mix cannabutter, regular butter, Graham cracker crumbs, powdered sugar and 1 cup creamy peanut butter until combined. Press evenly into bottom of 9×13 baking pan.

2.   In a saucepan and on medium heat, mix the chocolate chips, decarb seasoning and 4 tablespoons peanut butter until melted and combined.

3.   Spread the peanut butter mixture evenly on the crust and refrigerate for 2 hours.

4.   Cut into 1 inch squares before serving.

56. Chronic Apple Crisp

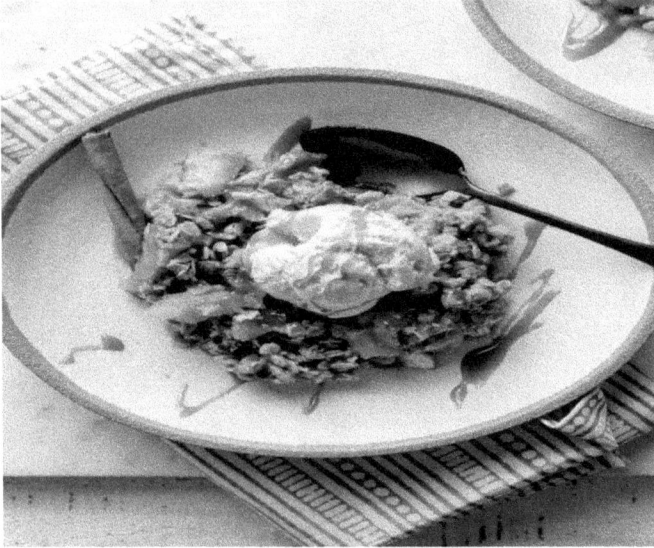

Ingredients:

10 cups apples, peeled, cored, and sliced 1 cup white sugar

1 cup + 1 tablespoon all-purpose flour 1 teaspoon ground cinnamon

½ cup water

1 cup quick cooking oats 1 cup brown sugar

¼ teaspoon baking powder

¼ teaspoon baking soda

½ cup cannabutter, melted 1 ounce cannabis tincture

Directions:

1. Heat oven to 350 degrees F. Spread apples evenly in 9×13 inch baking pan

2. In separate dish, mix cinnamon, 1 tablespoon flour and white sugar until combined. Sprinkle mix on apples. Pour water on apples.

3. In separate dish, mix oats, brown sugar, baking powder, baking soda, remaining flour, cannabutter and tincture until combined. Spread mixture

 evenly on top of apples'

4. Bake for 45 minutes. Serve warm.

57. Space Cake

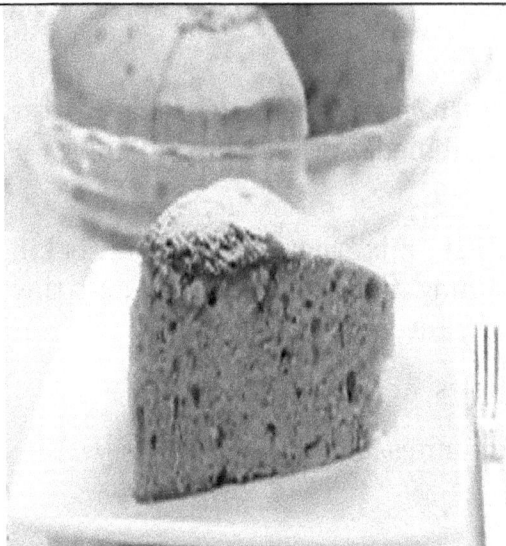

Ingredients:

1   ¼ cups of baking flour 200 CL. of milk

2   eggs

180 grams of sugar

¾ cup butter

8 grams of good (light) hash. (You can use Polm or Zero.)

Something to mix is always a nice touch. To give the cake a fresh taste: put 1 apple (sliced) in the cake. You can mix cacao (chocolate), a banana, vanilla (no ice cream!!)... nearly anything in it.

Directions:

1.   Preheat oven to 200 degrees c

2.   Put the butter in the microwave for about 20 seconds until it's a fat paste. Mix the hash with 4/5th of the butter. (Heat up the hash with a lighter and crumble it in the butter.) With the rest of the butter your fatten the baking form so you can get the cake out easy when it's done.

3.   Mix the butter (and hash), flour, eggs, milk and sugar (and the possible extra ingredient). Keep on mixing it for a few minutes until it's nice and smooth. If it's too dry: add a little milk. If there is too much liquid, add a little flour.

58. Cannabis Sugar Cookies

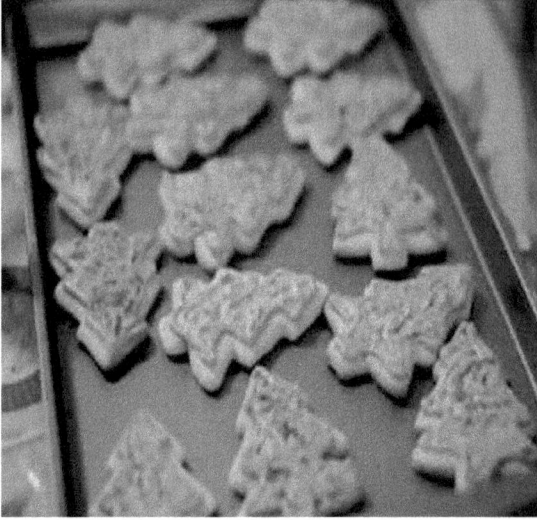

Ingredients:

1 cup of cannabis butter 1 cup brown sugar

1/2 cup white sugar 1 large egg

1   teaspoon vanilla

2   cups all-purpose flour

1/2 teaspoon of baking powder Pinch or two of salt

Directions:

1.   Preheat oven to

2.   Place the cannabis butter in a large bowl, and beat until it is very light and fluffy.

3.   Once fluffy, add sugar, a quarter cup at a time, continuing to vigorously beat the mix.

4.   Beat in the large egg and the vanilla flavoring.

5.   In a separate small bowl, mix together the baking powder, flour and the pinch of salt.

6.   Gradually beat the flour mix into the large bowl until completely mixed together.

7.   Divide the finished dough mixture into two halves, wrap each half in plastic wrap, and then refrigerate overnight.

8.   Roll each half with a rolling pin on a floured surface; the dough should have a thickness of about ? of an inch.

9.   Use a cookie cutter, any shape that you want, and then place the dough shapes onto a prepared cookie sheet at least 1 inch apart.

10.   Bake for 10-12 minutes, remove them from the oven when they look golden brown.

11.   Leave the cookies to cool before eating.

59. Strawberry Weed Muffins

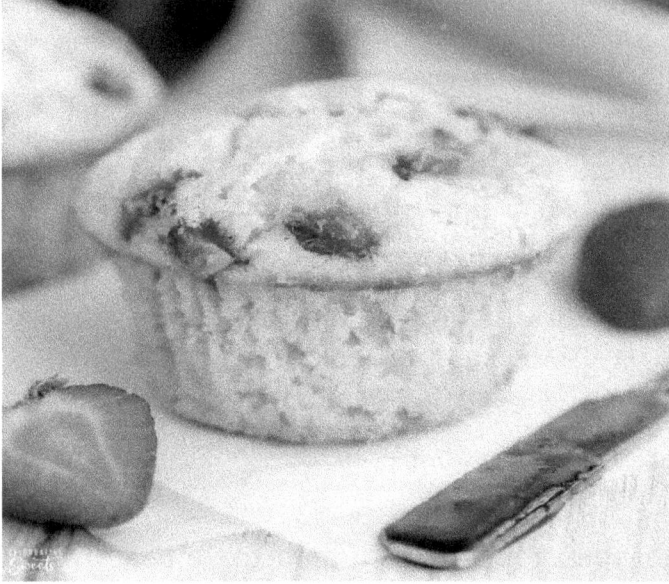

If you love strawberries, love muffins and love marijuana, then this recipe is your dream! It is also an easy recipe.

Ingredients:

1   cup of flour

1/2 cup of quick oats

2   teaspoons of baking powder 1/4 cup of sugar

1/2 teaspoon of salt 1 large egg

1/4 cup of cannabis butter 1 cup of milk

1 cup of fresh strawberries

Directions:

1.   Preheat oven to 380F-400F.

2.   Mix together the oats, flour, baking powder, sugar and salt in a large mixing bowl.

3.   In a smaller bowl, mix together the egg, milk and marijuana butter.

4.   Make a crater in the large bowl, and then pour in the liquid mix from the smaller bowl.

5.   Stir it up a little - don't stir until smooth - it should be lumpy.

6.   Carefully insert the strawberries deep into the mix; you can slice the strawberries into halves and quarters if you wish.

7.   Pour the mixture into a muffin tin, using muffin liners, make sure that you leave room in each muffin tin for them to rise. Your mix should fill about 75% of the capacity of the liners.

8.   Bake for 25-30 minutes in an oven.

9.   Leave to cool on a wire rack, and then enjoy!

60. Cannabombs

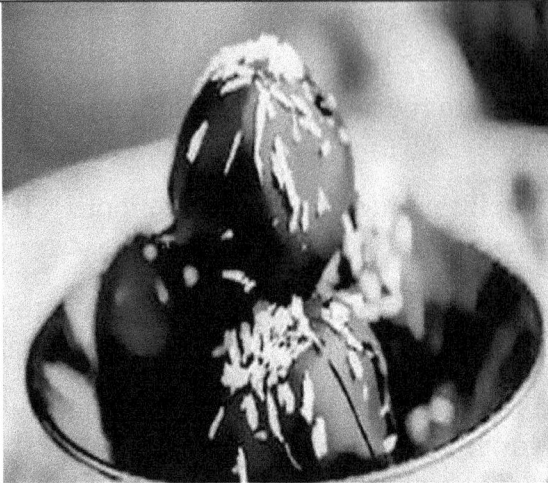

Items Need:

Medium sized pot Small ceramic dish Aluminum Foil

Oven bag (the kind used for cooking) Baking sheet

Candy thermometer Wax paper

Cheesecloth, optional (needed for larger quantities of herb)

*Double boiler

5 grams of hash or 14 grams of herb

(*If using a microwave chocolate, add the additional canna oil in the peanut butter and increase powder sugar accordingly - the double boiler pots are no longer required, unless making herb oil rather than hash oil.)

Ingredients:

2/3 cup peanut butter

2 – 2 ½ cups confectioners' sugar

½ teaspoon vanilla extract

1/2 cup butter and/or coconut oil – you can get away with less oil by using hash; this way, you won't dilute the peanut butter flavor quite so much with oil and sugar.

For Chocolate Coating:

Any hard, dark Bakers melting chocolate or chips, roughly ¾ – 1 cup. 2/3 teaspoon coconut hash oil (works better than the butter alternative, but use no other oil)

Paraffin/baking wax

Optional (recommended):

Lecithin powder

Optional (for "fuse"):

Thick, cotton cooking string, or white yarn Paraffin wax

Ceramic dish or a small home-made 'foil bowl'

Directions:

1. Preheat oven to 200 degrees F.

2. Cut 20 x 2 ½" sections of thick white string or yarn (you may need spares). Tie a small knot at one end of each string.

3. In oven, melt a small portion of paraffin wax in a small ceramic dish, takes only 2 – 3 minutes... it can be very carefully microwaved, or heated slowly on the stove-top, but it's MUCH, much safer and more controlled in the oven, and at a set temperature.

4.   Carefully remove the paraffin from the oven with a potholder - it will be very warm - so set it on a safe surface. Begin dipping the strings, tied end first, into the paraffin, coating the yarn well. If heated in the oven at 200, it should be cool enough to grab by the opposite end once dipped, to flip and coat the entire string. Be quick, or you'll be reheating your paraffin a few times! The wax helps keep the ball formed around the string, and it also prevents stray strands of string fiber from being eaten by you, your patients or your guests.

5.   Now you are ready to add your oils and lecithin.

6.   You can use a combination of oils, both for flavor and to create a varied oil 'vehicle' for cannabinoid bonding and availability, some thinner and some thicker. In the end, you want it to be a solid at room temp, so your canna balls aren't too soft, and the chocolate keeps its shape and thickness.

The additional liquid oils used in addition to the solids had previously been infused with herb.

7.   Ideally, you should be using butter and/or coconut oil, about 1 ½ tablespoons worth for your hash. If this is your primary or only canna oil source, you'll be adding an additional 2 tablespoons of softened butter to the peanut butter filling later on.

8.   And your double boiler, with your melted oils and lecithin over a low heat.

9.   (You can use slightly more oil, knowing that with this much herb, a small but noticeable quantity of oil will be left behind.)

10.   Cover tight with foil using the foil to seal the thermometer in place; keep between 180-200 degrees F, turning off the heat

periodically as it rises. This is what it looks like after about ten or so hours:

11.   Allow to cool somewhat, so it's only warm to the touch, and set up your cheesecloth.

12.   Now, you can begin straining.

13.   When using this much green for such a small amount of oil, I know there will be some potent material left within the herb that is worth keeping, so save and freeze the green for a future run, and use only the oil.

14.   However, knowing you'll be using a smaller amount, and if it was initially ground finely enough, you can choose to add it all directly to the peanut butter.

15.   Now with one (or both) of these oils, you're finally ready to make the peanut butter balls!

For the Peanut Butter Balls:

1.   In a mixing bowl, you'll be blending your peanut butter, vanilla and all your canna oil- except for roughly 2/3 teaspoon which will go in the chocolate - only if made with butter and/or coconut oil; otherwise, use it all in the peanut butter. If only using hash oil, remember to add a few tablespoons of additional butter at this point.

2.   Once that is done, you should have an oily peanut butter goo, and you're ready to begin mixing in your powdered sugar until it reaches a consistency that will hold shape and not crumble.

Making the Peanut Butter Centers Using the 'Fuse':

1.   Cover the base of a cookie sheet or baking pan with foil or wax paper.

2.   Take enough peanut butter filling, so that when rolled, it should create roughly a 1 1/4 – 1 1/2 inch diameter ball.

3.   Once it's balled up, insert the 'fuse' about half-way through the ball, KNOT-END FIRST, then gently squeeze and reform the ball making sure that it's stable.

4.   If you'd like, you can place them down gently but firmly on the foil or wax paper, just enough to create a 'flat' on the very base to keep them from rolling around.

5.   Having the fuse-knot in the center holds it in very snug, and prevents the fuse from slipping around and falling out, or crumbling the peanut butter; you can carefully bend the fuse so it looks decorative, or more 'cartoon- ish'.

6.   Pop the tray into the freezer for no longer than 20 minutes while you complete the following.

For Chocolate Coating:

1.   This can be as simple or tedious as you like. If you're not adept in the kitchen or familiar with tempering chocolate, I recommend using all your hash/canna oil in the peanut butter ball portion, disregard the double boiler, and use one of the newer, more simple microwavable melting chocolates, which are designed for easy, consistent use.

2.   Otherwise, you may be frustrated when the consistency fails, and it's more of a lumpy sauce than a coating.

3.   Using a double boiler pot, grab a handful of semisweet, dark and milk chocolate baking chips, concentrating on the dark and semisweet, and slowly melt them over the lowest heat possible.

4.   Once the chocolate is melted, add hash oil, blend and then begin shaving small amounts of paraffin into the chocolate. You will have to blend again, then drop a little on wax paper. Once it stays nice and solid, it's ready. Remove from heat.

5.   If you choose to make your own chocolate coat but without adding additional canna oil, there is no need for the paraffin; just temper as usual,

and they will be much shinier this way. Remember the smaller and taller the pot, the easier it will be to use as a coat.

6.   Remove your peanut butter balls from the freezer (or the refrigerator, if you waited longer than 20 minutes), and grab them one at a time by the fuse.

7.   Quickly dunk each ball in the cooling chocolate, and place on your wax paper. A new sheet can be used, or you can carefully return each ball to the last sheet.

8.   The cold temperature of the peanut butter ball will rapidly solidify the cooling chocolate. This is why it's best to work fast and use the freezer rather than the fridge for the ball; the outer edge becomes colder than it can in the fridge without allowing the center to become frozen (which can cause crumbling/cracking in the center around the fuse when dunked into the warm chocolate).

9.   After dunking each ball, take a spoon. Using the excess chocolate, place a small drop on the end of each fuse... now they're lit.

10.   Pop them in the freezer, and you're done!

61. Weed Banana Bread

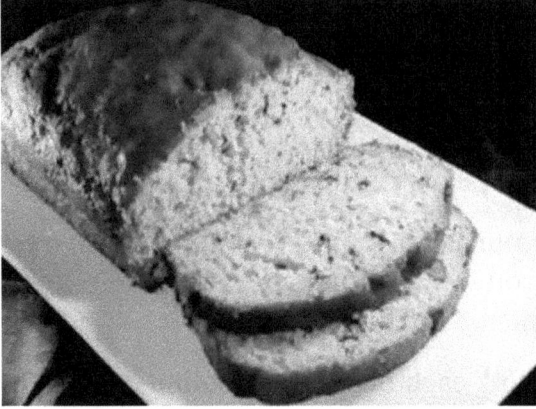

Prep Time: 5 minutes Cook Time: 50-60 minutes Serves:10-12

Recommended Dosage: 3 tablespoons cannabutter

Ingredients:

2 cups flour 1/2 cup sugar

1 teaspoon baking soda 1/2 teaspoon salt

1   1/2 cups mashed ripe bananas

1/4 cup honey or agave nectar (lower glycemic index) 1/4 cup sour cream

2   large eggs, lightly beaten 6 tablespoons melted butter 1 teaspoon vanilla

1 1/4 cups toasted and chopped pecans

Directions:

1.   Preheat oven to 350 degrees F. Grease and flour a 9X5 inch loaf pan and set aside.

2.   In a medium bowl, combine the flour, sugar, baking soda and salt; then, mix well and set aside. In a large bowl, mix the mashed bananas, honey, sour cream, eggs, melted butter and vanilla.

3.   Lightly fold the dry ingredients into the wet ingredients, mixing only until incorporated. Stir in the chopped pecans. Batter will be lumpy.

4.   Pour batter into prepared pan and bake for 50-60 minutes, or until a tester comes out clean.

5.   Cool in pan for 5 minutes, then transfer to a wire rack to cool completely.

62. Mint Cnnabis Browies

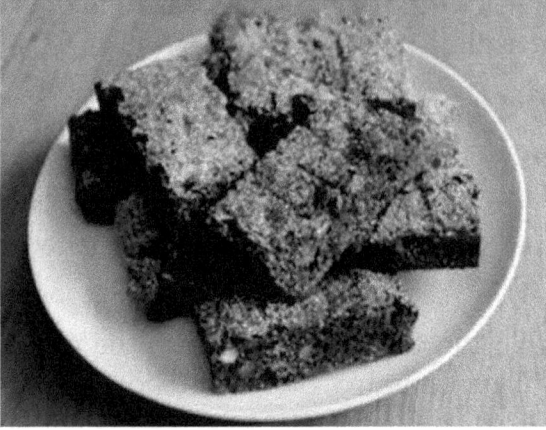

These delicious cannabrownies deliver a potent punch AND give you that satisfying chocolate/mint combination. Don't forget these for your Christmas party.

Ingredients:

1 cup cannabutter

6 ounces unsweetened chocolate 2 cups sugar

1 teaspoon baking powder 1½ teaspoons vanilla

½ teaspoon salt 1½ cups flour

1 cup walnuts or pecans, finely ground

1 1/2 ounces bag Hershey's mint chocolate chips 4 eggs

Directions:

1.   Preheat oven to

2.   In a medium saucepan, melt cannabutter and unsweetened chocolate over low heat, stirring constantly. Remove from heat and let cool.

3.   Grease 9×13 inch pan and set aside. Stir sugar into cooled chocolate mixture in saucepan. Beat eggs, and add slowly to chocolate mixture. Stir in vanilla.

4.   In a bowl, stir together the flour, baking soda and salt.

5.   Add flour mixture to chocolate mixture until combined. Stir in nuts and mint chocolate chips. Spread the batter in the prepared pan.

6.   Bake for 30 minutes. Cool on wire rack before storing.

63. Poppy-Pot Cake

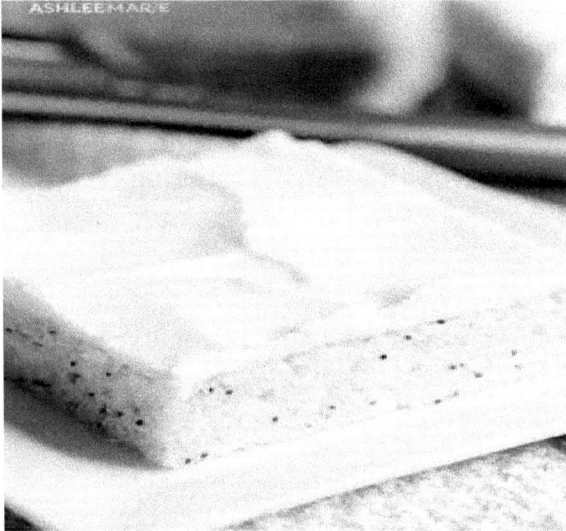

Ingredients:

For Cake :

1 3/4 cups cannaflour

1/2 teaspoon baking powder 1/2 teaspoon baking soda 1/8 teaspoon salt

1/2 cup unsalted cannabutter, softened 1 1/4 cups sugar

3 eggs

1 cup creme fraiche

3   tablespoons poppy seeds 1/2 teaspoon almond extract

For Frosting:

4   ounces cream cheese, softened 2/3 cup powdered sugar

1 cup creme fraiche

1   teaspoon finely grated lemon peel 1/8 teaspoon almond extract

Directions:

1.   Preheat oven to 350 degrees F. Spray bottom of a 9-inch square pan with nonstick cooking spray.

2.   In a medium bowl, stir together cannaflour, baking powder, baking soda and salt.

3.   In a large bowl, beat butter at a medium speed for 30 seconds, until creamy. Add sugar, beat for 5 minutes or until light, creamy and fluffy. Add eggs one at a time, beating until blended.

4.   At low speed, beat in flour mixture in 3 parts alternately, with 1 cup creme fraiche, beginning and ending with flour mixture. Beat in poppy seeds and 1/2 teaspoon almond extract.

5.   Spoon and spread batter into pan (It will be very thick). Bake 35-40 minutes or until dark golden brown and toothpick inserted in center comes out clean. Cool completely on wire rack.

6.   Right before serving, in another large bowl, beat cream cheese and powdered sugar at low speed until smooth. Slowly beat in 1 cup creme fraiche until blended. Increase speed to medium; beat frosting until firm, but do not let stiff peaks form. Beat in lemon peel and 1/8 teaspoon almond extract.

7.   Spread frosting over cake. Store in refrigerator.

64. Purple Kush Cake

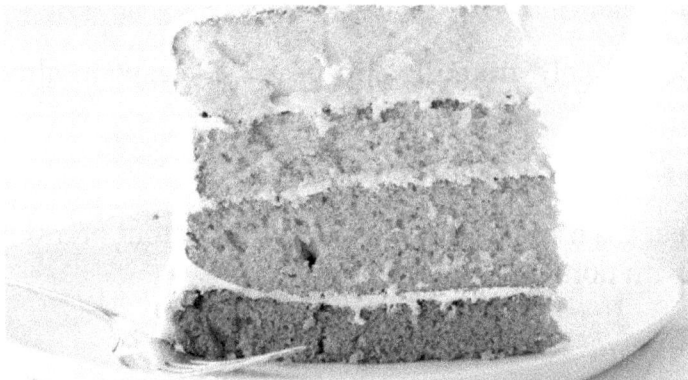

You love Purple Kush? Well, you're going to go insane for this cake. The best chocolate cake recipe ever!

Ingredients:

¾ cup THC oil1

18.25-ounce Betty Crocker Super Moist Dark Chocolate Mix 3 eggs

2   cups cold milk

One 16-ounce tub Betty Crocker Rich & Creamy Vanilla Frosting

Directions:

1.   Preheat oven to 400 degrees F.

2.   Mix together the cake referencing the package directions. Use the infused oil instead of cooking oil and mix it with the eggs and water.

3.   Pour the cake mixture into 2 evenly sized pans, and bake for 30 minutes or until a knife comes out of the cake cleans.

4.   Mix the frosting until smooth and spread a layer over the top of one cake. Put the other cake on top to create a cake sandwich. Now smother the entire cake in frosting and enjoy!

65. Fire Crackers

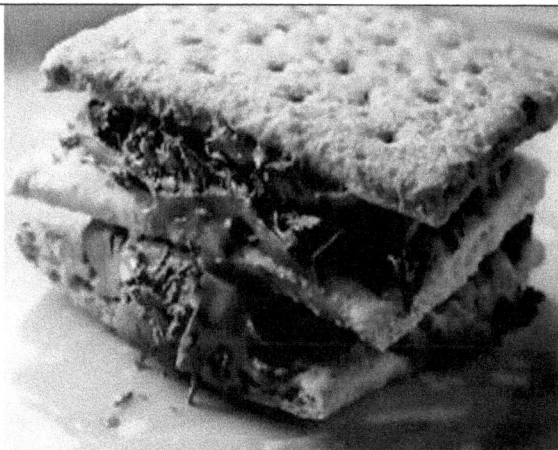

Ingredients:

Weed: A bowl (0.3 to 2 grams) per firecracker. The amount you will want to use depends on your tolerance. Use the same amount you would normally smoke. We estimate this at about half a gram all the way up to 2 grams for those who pack tight and smoke to great heights for each firecracker you are going to make.

We are going to eat our firecrackers for medical purposes so we are choosing a medical strain, Harlequin. It has a floral taste like a bouquet of flowers, perfect for our peanut butter and Nutella cookie sandwiches.

Saltine crackers: Choose your favorite cracker. Since you will be adding peanut butter, you may want to choose a cracker with less sugar so that it doesn't taste so much like a cookie. You also want a cracker, a Graham or Ritz cracker, that can withstand a little baking without coming apart.

Peanut Butter: Choose your favorite peanut butter. You may want to go organic with less sugar. It's important that the peanut butter has mostly natural peanut oil rather than soybean oil, although soybean oil will still work.

Nutella: You can use Nutella only or peanut butter only or mix them. Nutella is a hazelnut and chocolate spread. It is mostly hazel nut but also has cocoa in it. Some people love the taste.

Directions:

1.   Preheat oven to 250 degrees F.

2.   Decarb your weed. The first thing you want to do is decarb your weed. Decarboxylating your weed is going to convert inactive THCA to potent THC. Now, take your gram or more of weed, and place it in the oven for ten minutes. Now your Harlequin weed is activated, full of THC and CBD. It will look a bit brown and toasted. It should smell really dank, pungent, and delicious.

3.   Spread peanut butter and Nutella on your cracker. You may want to put peanut butter on one cracker and Nutella on another.

4.   Add 0.3 to 2 grams of decarbed weed into the peanut butter on the cracker. Mix it in. The oil in the peanut butter is going to extract the cannabinoids, so make sure you mix it in good into the peanut butter side because it has the most reliable oils. Now, put one cracker on top of the other.

5.   Wrap your sandwiched crackers in tin foil. The foil will protect your cannabinoids from evaporating away.

6.   Raise the temperature to 300 degrees F. Bake your weed firecrackers in a toaster oven for 15 minutes.

7.   Remove. Let it cool on your plate.

8.   Your firecracker is ready to be consumed. It's that simple...you've made your easiest weed edible to make. But don't let the ease of baking fool you, this edible is as powerful as the weed you put in it, so be mindful of how much weed you have used and how much THC it has. Respect the weed and you will have a great time.

66. Cinnamon Pecan Sandies

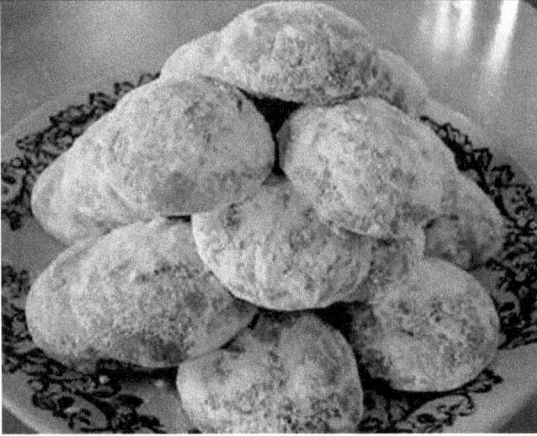

Ingredients:

1   cup ground pecans 1 cup cannabutter

2   cups all-purpose flour

½ teaspoon baking powder 1 tablespoon vanilla extract 1 cup natural brown sugar 2 teaspoons cinnamon

½ cup sifted powdered sugar

Directions:

1.   Preheat oven to 352 degrees F.

2.   Cream the cannabutter and sugar together in a mixing bowl until smooth. While creaming, add in the vanilla. Sift together the flour and baking powder and gradually add it to your mixing bowl. Add the chopped pecans. Cover the dough and chill for 3-4 hours.

3.   Remove the dough from the refrigerator and roll it into golf-sized balls before gently flattening them in your hand and placing them on an ungreased cookie sheet.

4.   Bake for about 20 minutes or until slightly firm and golden. Remove from the oven and gently placing them on a cooling rack.

5.   Combine the sifted powdered sugar and cinnamon and dust them with the mixture. Allow them to completely cool to avoid crumbling. Enjoy!

67. Cheech and Chong's Chocolate Cake

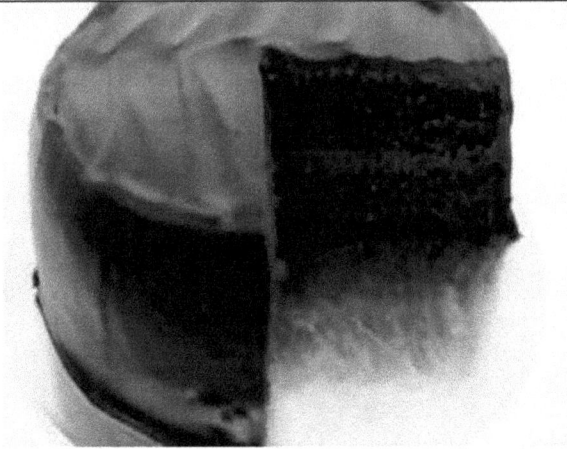

This is a chocolatey delight that will be sure to have you coming back for more.

Ingredients:

1 cup dark chocolate 1 cup cannabutter

1 1/2 cups caster sugar, plus an extra pinch 6 eggs, separated into yolks and whites 1/2 cup ground almonds

3/4 cup soft white breadcrumbs 1/8 cup plain flour

4 teaspoons vanilla essence

For the Icing:

3/8 cup cocoa powder 1 cup icing sugar

2/3 cup butter

3/4 cup caster sugaz 6 tablespoons water

Directions:

For the Space Cake:

1.   Preheat the oven to 325 degrees F. Grease and line a 10 inch round cake tin.

2.   Melt the chocolate in a double boiler or in a bowl placed over a pan of boiling water.

3.   Cream the cannabis butter with 1 1/2 cups sugar until pale and softened.

4.   Gradually beat in the egg yolks and stir in the almonds. Fold in the cool melted chocolate, breadcrumbs, flour and vanilla essence.

5.   In a separate bowl, whip the egg whites with a pinch of sugar until stiff but not dry. Fold into the cake mixture and pour into the prepared cake tin.

6.   Bake for 1 hour until firm to the touch.

For the Icing:

1.   Sieve the cocoa and icing sugar into a bowl.

2.   Warm the butter, sugar and water in a microwave or double boiler and simmer until the sugar has dissolved.

3.   Add the liquid to the dry mixture and combine until thickened.

4.   Spread the icing over the cooled hash cake.

68. Twice-Cooked Popcorn Bars

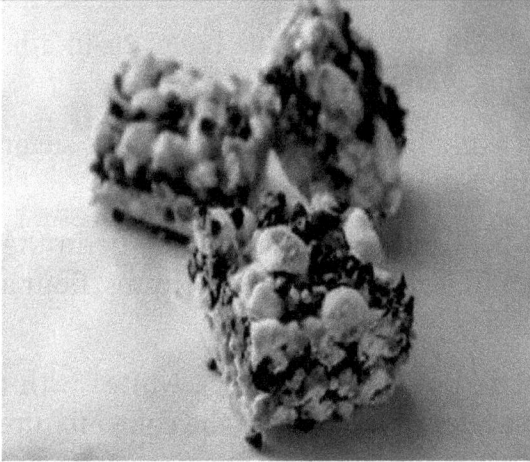

Yield: 9-12 portions

Ingredients:

8 tablespoons cannabutter

6 cups marshmallows or mini marshmallows, don't count, it's a bag! 5 tablespoons peanut butter

7-8 cups popped caramel corn or popcorn 1 cup peanuts, chopped

1 cup mini chocolate chips

For Topping:

½ cup mini marshmallows

½ cup mini chocolate chips

Directions:

1.   Heat oven to 350 degrees F.

2.   Cover the bottom of a 9-inch square pan with parchment paper.

3.   In a large saucepan melt the butter. Add the marshmallows and stir until fully melted. Stir in the peanut butter.

4.   Add the popcorn and mix until evenly coated. Spread half the mixture into prepared pan. With damp clean hands, press the popcorn down and try

to make even thickness. Sprinkle with the peanuts and the chocolate chips.

5.   Press the remaining popcorn mixture on top of the peanuts and chocolate.

6.   Sprinkle with the remaining marshmallows and chocolate chips, and place in the oven for 5-7 minutes.

7.   Allow to cool and then chill in refrigerator before cutting.

69. Peppermint Buddha Bark

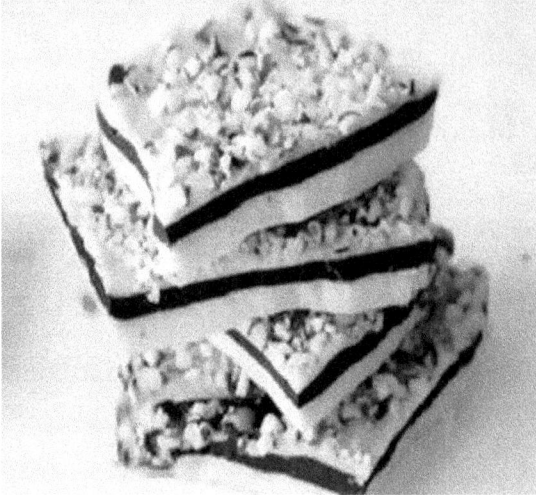

Peppermint bark is a delicious, festive treat that pleases just about everyone who tries it. This medicated recipe perfectly features the peppermint flavor that many of us have grown accustomed to associating with the holiday season, as well as both white and semisweet chocolate layers.

Ingredients:

12 ounces white chocolate

6 ounces semisweet chocolate

4 tablespoons cannabis-infused coconut oil

½ teaspoon peppermint extract 3 candy canes (crushed)

Directions:

1.   Line a 9×9 inch baking pan with some parchment paper or aluminum foil, making sure to wrap the foil over the sides of the pan, and smooth out any wrinkles as you go. This step will ensure a quick clean up and will also allow for the peppermint bark to easily pop off the pan when it comes time to break it into individual pieces.

2.   Melt together the semisweet chocolate chips and the white chocolate chips. To do this, create a double boiler using a heat-safe bowl and a saucepan filled with water. Choose a bowl that fits snugly over the top of

the saucepan (Do not use a bowl that sits precariously on top of the pot). You also want to ensure that the bottom of the bowl does not touch the water or you risk burning the chocolate.

3.   As an aside, this recipe uses 3 layers of chocolate for the bark (white, semisweet, white). Feel free to switch up the quantities of the chocolate and reverse the layering (semisweet, white, semisweet) if you so please!

4.   Bring the water in the saucepan to a simmer, and place the heat-safe bowl containing your white chocolate chips over the sauce pan.

5.   Melt the white chocolate chips until they're smooth.

6.   Add in 4 tablespoons of cannabis-infused coconut oil and the ½ teaspoon of peppermint extract.

7.   Stir until both oils have fully dissolved into the white chocolate. Aside from medicating the dish, the coconut oil will also create a nice shine in the bark and allow it to have a good "snap" when breaking up the pieces.

8.   Once the melted white chocolate is smooth again, pour half of it into the prepped pan. Tilt the pan after you pour in half of the melted white chocolate to ensure an even coating/first layer.

9.   Place the pan in the refrigerator and allow the first layer of chocolate to harden completely, roughly 30 minutes or so.

10.   While your first layer of bark is setting, repeat the above steps in order to prepare a second double boiler for your semi-sweet chocolate chips.

11.   Once your semisweet chocolate chips are completely melted, remove the bowl from the double boiler.

12.   Take the pan containing the first layer of white chocolate from the refrigerator and proceed to pour the entire bowl of melted semisweet chocolate chips over the first layer. It is extremely important that the initial layer of white chocolate is completely hardened, as introducing the second layer will cause them to mix if this is not the case.

13.   Spread the second layer of semisweet chocolate chips evenly throughout the pan using a spatula or baker's knife.

14.   Place the pan back into the refrigerator as you wait for the second layer of chocolate to set, again roughly 30 minutes or so.

15.   When the second layer of chocolate has set, add the third and final layer of white chocolate on top of the semisweet layer. Spread this third layer evenly with a spatula.

16.   Place the candy canes into a Ziploc bag and proceed to crush them into tiny pieces using the back of a ladle or a rolling pin.

17.   Sprinkle the crushed candy canes on top of the third and final layer of white chocolate covering the entire surface, and then place the pan back into the refrigerator until the bark is completely set (30 minutes to 1 hour).

18.   When ready to eat, remove the bark from the refrigerator and pull up on the sides of the aluminum foil – the bark should lift right out of the pan!

19.   Break the bark into individual pieces, and either package them up to give as a gift, or serve them to your guests immediately!

70. Almond Lemon Bars

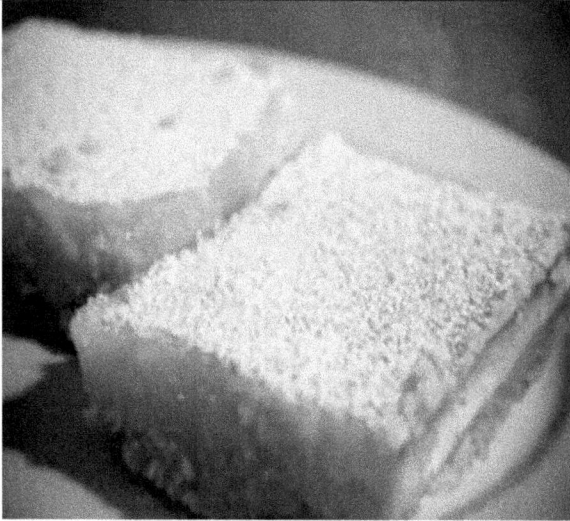

Lemon bars remind me of spring time. They are bright, tart and sweet- creamy-goodness, all wrapped up into one delicious dessert. This medicated recipe features classic lemon bars topped with sugary, sliced almonds. Send your taste buds on a trip to Flavor Town with this citrus dessert.

Yield: 32 lemon bars

Ingredients:

1/4 cup granulated sugar

3/4 cup cannabis-infused butter (softened) 1 teaspoon lemon zest

2 cups all-purpose flour 1/4 teaspoon table salt

For Lemon Bar Batter:

6 large eggs

2 cups sugar

1/4 cup chopped, crystallized ginger 1/2 cup all-purpose flour

1 teaspoon baking powder 2 tablespoons lemon zest 2/3 cup fresh lemon juice

For Almond Mixture:

3/4 cup flour 1/2 cup sugar

1/4 teaspoon salt

1/4 cup cannabis-infused butter (melted) 1/2 cup sliced almonds

Optional garnishes: a dusting of powdered sugar, whipped cream, etc.

Directions:

For Lemon Bar Crust:

1.   Preheat your oven to 350 degrees F.

2.   Using a standing or hand-held electric mixer, beat 1/4 cup of sugar, 3/4 cup of softened cannabis-infused butter and 1 teaspoon of lemon zest at medium speed for 2 minutes or until the mixture is creamy.

3.   In a separate large bowl, combine 2 cups of flour and 1/4 teaspoon of salt. Gradually add the dry goods (flour and salt) to the creamed butter, sugar and eggs. Mix well until everything is thoroughly combined.

4.   After the dough crust is mixed, prep a 9x13 inch baking dish with some nonstick cooking spray. Place the empty, greased dish into the refrigerator to chill for at least 15 minutes prior to baking.

5.   Remove the dish from the refrigerator, and press the dough into the pan until you create a uniform layer. (Don't miss the corners!)

6.   Bake the crust for 15 to 20 minutes in your preheated oven or until lightly browned.

7.   Remove the crust from the oven and reduce the oven temperature to 325 degrees F.

8.   Let the crust sit to the side for now.

For Lemon Bar Batter:

1.   Whisk together the 6 eggs and 2 cups of sugar.

2.   In a food processor or blender, pour in the 1/2 cup of flour along with the 1/4 cup of crystallized ginger. Pulse the two ingredients together until fully combined. Proceed to pour the flour and ginger blend into a medium size bowl.

3.   Stir 1 teaspoon of baking powder into the flour and ginger blend.

4.   Slowly add batches of the flour and ginger blend to the bowl containing the eggs and sugar.

5.   Whisk in the lemon juice and 2 tablespoons of lemon zest until fully combined and smooth.

6.   Pour the lemon bar batter over the cooled crust, shimmying and jiggling the dish to allow any air bubbles to escape.

7.   Bake the lemon bars in your preheated oven for 15 to 20 minutes or until the lemon filling has just barely set.

8.   Remove the lemon bars from the oven and place them to the side for now.

For Sliced Almond Mixture:

1.   Stir the remaining 3/4 cup flour, 1/2 cup of sugar and 1/4 teaspoon of salt together in a small bowl.

2.   Pour in the 1/4 cup of melted cannabis-infused butter, and stir the ingredients until they're well blended.

3.   Add the 1/2 cup of sliced almonds, and stir once more.

4.   Sprinkle the almond and sugar mixture over the hot lemon bars, and then place the lemon bars back into the oven for an additional 20 to 25 minutes or until they're lightly golden in color.

5.   Remove the lemon bars from the oven and allow them to cool in the baking dish on top of a wire cooling rack for at least 1 hour.

6.   Cut your lemon bars into individual squares, and serve immediately with a dash of powdered sugar, if you so please.

7.   Enjoy.

71.Weed Macaroons

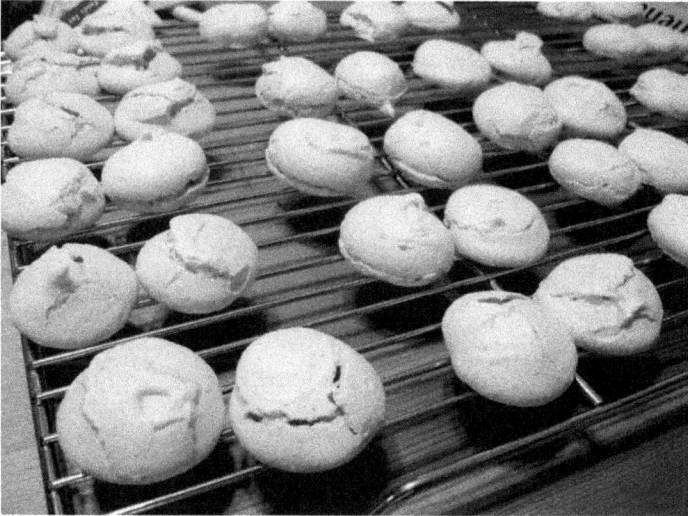

Have you ever had coconut macaroons? They are simply divine little treats. For those of you who prefer edibles instead of smoking, here is a delightful recipe for marijuana with coconut macaroons that you can't say no to.

Ingredients:

1   1/3 cups of flaked coconut 1/3 cup of sugar

2   tablespoons flour Pinch of salt

Egg whites of 2 eggs Vanilla extract

2 tablespoons of cannabis butter Baking chocolate or chocolate chips Chopped nuts (optional)

Directions:

1.   Preheat oven to 325 degrees F and grease a large biscuit sheet or tray.

2.   Combine together in a bowl the coconut, sugar, flour and salt. Use your hands to mix them well and break off any large

lumps of coconut or flour. Once they are mixed well, set them aside and move on to the egg whites.

3.   Crack the eggs and separate the egg whites from the yolks into a bowl. Then add half a teaspoon of vanilla extract to the egg whites.

4.   Whip the egg whites very fast with a whisk or an electric hand mixer to get a nice, shiny and frothy mixture. It is important to do this step well; otherwise, the egg whites will run out of the meringue while it's cooking.

5.   Add the whisked egg whites and vanilla extract mixture to the dry coconut and flour mix and combine the dry and wet ingredients together by tossing them with wooden spoons as it gives them a light and fluffy look.

6.   Once the mixture is ready, put one tablespoon scoops of the mixture on the greased biscuit tray. You will get about a dozen scoops from this mixture.

7.   Put the tray into the preheated oven for 15 to 18 minutes until the macaroons are golden brown. Keep an eye on them so they don't burn on the bottom.

For the Marijuana Chocolate:

1.   For this you will need to prepare a double boiler with a pan filled with water and a glass bowl placed above it. Bring the water to a boil and then add the cannabis butter to the bowl and let it melt.

2.   Once the butter has melted, start adding the chocolate to the cannabis butter in the bowl. As it melts, incorporate it gently with the butter using a spatula to get a glossy mixture. You can use any chocolate of your choice – milk, dark or white chocolate.

3.   Check on the macaroons; they should be done by now. Take them out of the oven and let them cool for a few minutes before transferring them to a cooling wire rack.

4.   Meanwhile, the chocolate sauce should be ready. Keep the flame on simmer so the sauce remains liquid. Once the macaroons have cooled down they are ready to be dipped in the marijuana chocolate sauce. Hold them from the bottom and dip the tops gently into the sauce. If you want the macaroons to be stronger you can double dip them in the marijuana chocolate again.

5.   You can top them off with chopped nuts of your choice and voila! They are ready to be eaten.

72. Weed Cotton Candy

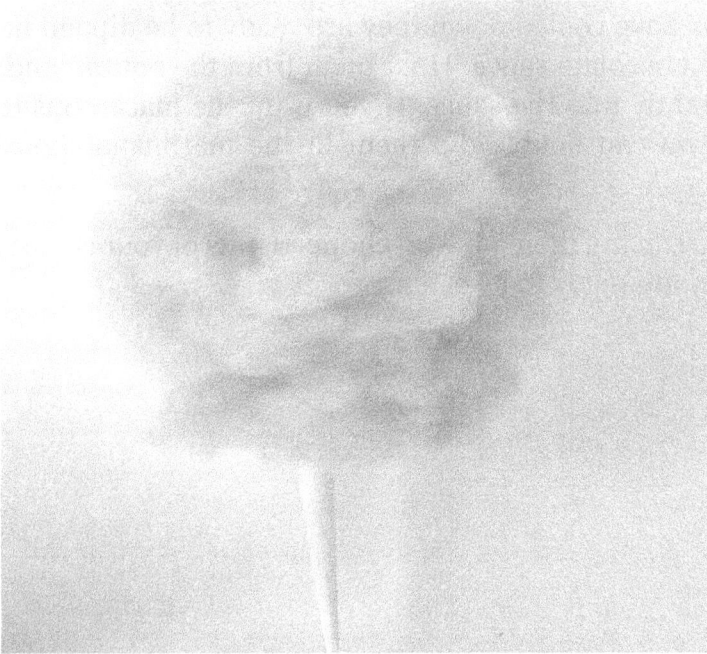

Items Needed:

Mortar and pestle Cotton candy machine Lollipop sticks Measuring scoop

Ingredients:

2-3   weed candies

2 scoops flossine

Directions:

1.   Crush 2-3 weed candies using the mortar and pestle. Add flossine to the powder and crush it again. It's important to ensure that the powdered candy is smooth and fine.

2.   Next, the powdered mixture needs to be spun into candy with the help of the cotton candy machine. To use the candy machine correctly, it's important to set it on a steady, flat and smooth surface. Also, ensure that the machine is placed at a safe height, away from the reach of children and pets. Once the necessary precautions are taken, the cotton candy machine is set to be used.

3.   Once in place, turn on the candy machine's mortar and fill the floss head with about 2 scoops of the candy-flossine mixture. You might want to make sure that you are not filling more than 90% of the floss head.

4.   The secret to spinning the perfect cotton candy is getting the details right, starting from the very beginning until the very last step.

5.   After about 30-40 seconds of turning on the heat, you will see threads of the candy forming in the machine. Dip a lollipop stick inside and gather the cotton candy by twirling the stick around. Do not rotate the stick itself, but move it in a circular motion instead. Avoid touching the edges and turn off the machine once the cotton candy is done.

6.   After a couple of trials, you'll be able to spin the perfect weed cotton candy, much to the amazement of those around you!

73. Cannabis Coffee Cake

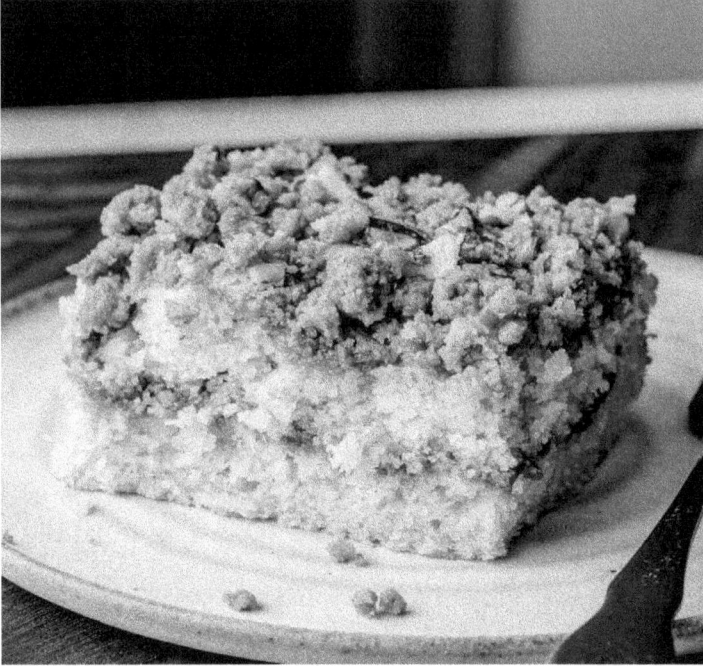

Coffee has never tasted better when accompanied by this delicious cannabis coffee cake, and it is a great way to start your day.

Ingredients:

2 ¼ cups flour

1 package active yeast 2/3 cup milk

6 tablespoons vegetable shortening 6 tablespoons sugar

1/4 teaspoon salt 1 egg

1/2 cup sliced almonds

1 ½ tablespoons cannabis butter (melted)

Directions:

1.   Preheat oven to 375 degrees F.

2.   In a medium mixing bowl, add I cup flour and the package of active yeast. Set it aside.

3.   In a medium saucepan, add the milk, vegetable shortening and 4 tablespoons of sugar. Heat the pan and stir occasionally. Once the vegetable shortening has softened, remove the mixture from the heat and add the contents to the yeast and flour mixture.

4.   Add the egg and beat ingredients for one minute in an electric mixture. Remove mixture from the sides of the bowl by scraping it and continue to

beat the mixture for another 3 to 5 minutes. Slowly stir in the rest of the flour to form pliant dough.

5.   Use the nonstick cooking spray to grease the baking pan. If you do not have cooking spray, grease it conventionally. Place the cake mixture into the baking pan. Sprinkle the top of the dough with sliced almonds and the remaining sugar. Cover it with a clean and damp dish cloth, and set aside for one hour to allow the dough to rise. Will normally take an hour or so.

6.   Remove the dish cloth and drizzle the risen dough with melted cannabis butter. Bake for 17 to 20 minutes. Allow to cool. Slice, eat and feel heavenly.

74. Weed Popsicles

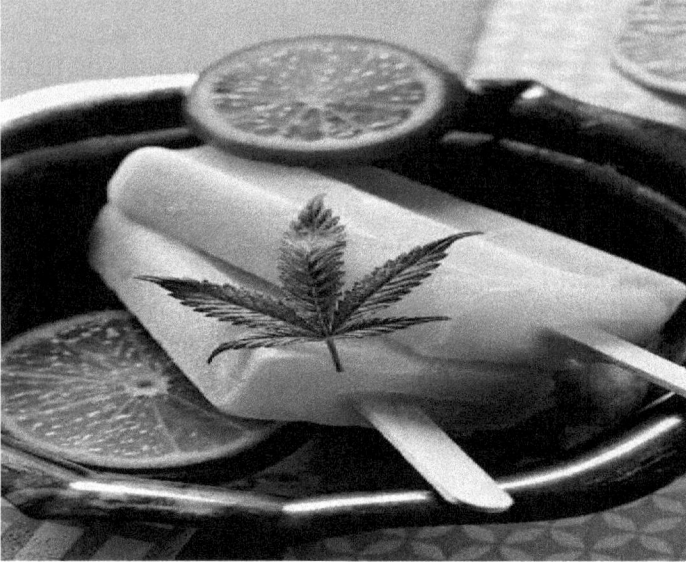

Have you ever thought about mixing your medical marijuana into a frozen treat, but were not sure on how to go about it? Well, here is a recipe you can use to create some amazingly delicious medicated popsicles. Trust me...this is a popsicle that you are going to want to make again and again and again.

Ingredients:

2   mangos, peeled and in chunks

2 cups of your favorite vanilla yogurt 4 tablespoons cream of coconut

**2-3 tablespoons of medicated coconut oil 3 tablespoons coconut sugar

2 teaspoons coconut extract

If you do not like the taste of coconut, then you are more than welcome to use any substitute.

Directions:

1.   There are actually only four easy steps you need to follow to get yourself on your way to enjoying your popsicles, and those are as follows :

2.   Place all of your ingredients into your blender.

3.   Puree them until they are smooth.

4.   Pour them into popsicle molds.

5.   Freeze them.

6.   And you are done! Once you are sure that your popsicles are nice and frozen, you can take them out of their mold and enjoy them! There has

never been a simpler way to create an awesome medicated treat that you can enjoy on a hot summer day.

** For Medicated Coconut Oil:

Ingredients:

2 cups of coconut oil

1 ounce of medical marijuana

Directions:

1.   Making some medicated coconut oil for you to cook with is easy! All you have to do is place some coconut oil and cannabis in a pan, and simmer for 20 or so minutes. Once you are done, separate the leftover plant matter from the oil with a strainer. Make sure to get every last drop out of the plant matter so you do not waste anything.

2.   Keep the heat low so that you do not mess with the THC levels of your cannabis. There have been a few studies that show that boiling cannabis can eliminate a lot of the THC which can ruin it for cooking or anything else. So, it is best to keep an eye on your cannabis while it is simmering.

3.   Overall, this is a very simple recipe that you and any of your friends will love. As stated before, it is a completely customizable recipe, so you can change out any of the ingredients for something else. The possibilities are endless!

4.   So go and create your weed popsicle today, and see what amazing frozen treat you make!

75. Cannabis Granola

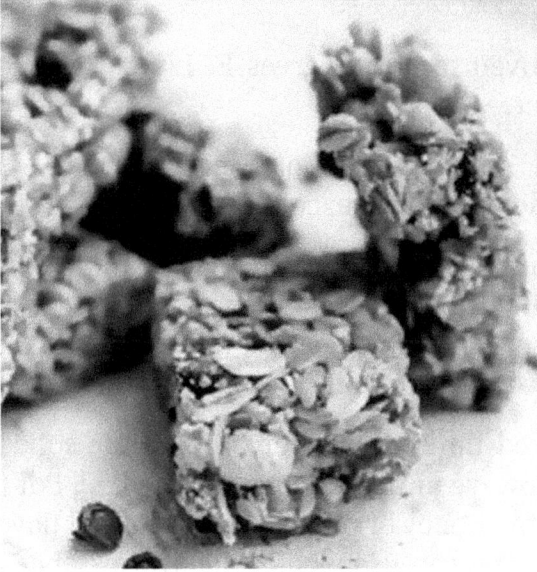

Weed granola bars are usually made using cannabis butter or weed-infused coconut oil. Here is a quick and easy recipe of weed granola bars that you can try at home.

Ingredients:

½ cup of marijuana-infused coconut oil 3 cups of oatmeal

1 cup of chopped nuts of your choice Berries or fruits of your choice

1 teaspoon baking soda

½ cup of brown flaxseed meal

1 ½ teaspoons of cinnamon powder

½ cup of honey or maple syrup Any optional flavorings

A pinch of salt

Directions:

1.   Preheat oven to 300 degrees F. Line a biscuit tray with parchment paper.

2.   Mix the oatmeal, chopped nuts, flaxseed meal and cinnamon powder together - except the salt.

3.   Mix them up nicely with your hands and set the mixture aside. The ground flaxseed is being used because there is marijuana infused-oil in this recipe, and the ground flaxseed will help absorb any of the extra oil.

4.   If the weed-infused coconut oil is in the solid state, just heat it in a microwave until it melts into liquid oil. Put the oil into a bowl and add the honey or maple syrup, salt and flavorings to it and mix it well. You can use whatever flavor essences you want depending on your taste - for instance, vanilla, strawberry, pineapple etc.

5.   Once the liquid mixture is ready, you can add it to the dry mix that you prepared earlier. Toss and mix everything using spoons, and put the combined mixture into the tray lined with parchment paper. Spread the entire mixture evenly in the tray without pressing down on it.

6.   Pop this mix into the preheated oven for about 20 to 30 minutes, and let it cook until it is golden brown. You may check on it after 10 minutes and take it out to stir the mixture around a bit. Then put the mixture back into the oven for 15 to 20 minutes more until you find it becoming golden brown.

7.   Take it out and stir in any fresh or dry fruits you like such as berries or other fruit segments. Once it cools a bit, you can shape the granola mix into bars with your hands. Once the bars are done, leave them to cool properly, and your weed granola bars

are done! You can store them easily in boxes or bags; they make a great breakfast or snack.

76. Baked Backlava

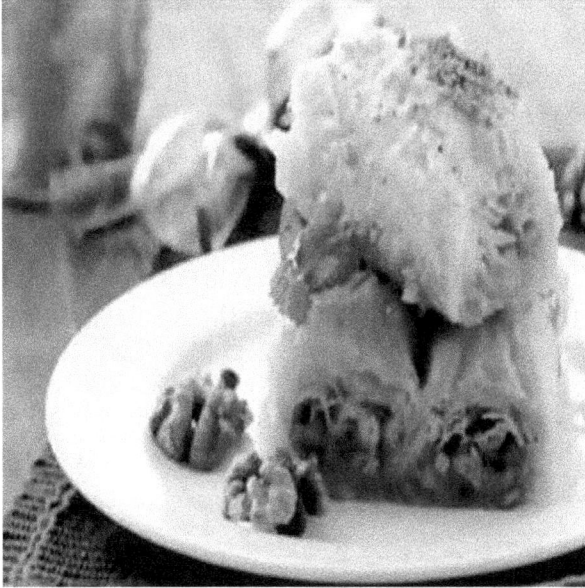

Try these delicious and delightfully gooey snacks. They will not only impress your friends, but they are sure to come back another time for the kick again. Edibles have never tasted this good!

Ingredients:

1 1/2 pounds walnuts, chopped 2 cups sugar

1/2 teaspoon nutmeg 3 teaspoons cinnamon 3 sticks canna butter

16 ounces phyllo dough 1 1/2 cups water

1 1/2 teaspoons Lemon Juice 2 cups honey

1/2 teaspoon vanilla

Directions:

1.   Preheat oven to 300 degrees F.

2.   Set aside 2 tablespoons of the cannabutter. With the remaining butter, grease a 10×15 inch baking dish.

3.   Take 10 sheets of phyllo dough, coat each with a good layer of butter and place them in the baking pan.

4.   Mix together the walnuts with one cup of sugar, and pour this evenly into the pan over the phyllo dough sheets.

5.   Take another five layers of phyllo dough, butter them and then place them in the pan as well. Bake the dough for 50 minutes.

6.   While this is baking, take a saucepan and mix the leftover sugar with the spices, vanilla, water and lemon; cook until the mixture is syrupy. Add honey and heat for a minute. Remove from heat.

7.   Cut the baklava into 2 by 2 inch squares or any other shape you want and then pour the syrup over them.

8.   Now, have patience- set aside for two days so as to allow the honey to permeate. You are now ready for this spicy canna treat.

77. Butterscotch Canna-Pops

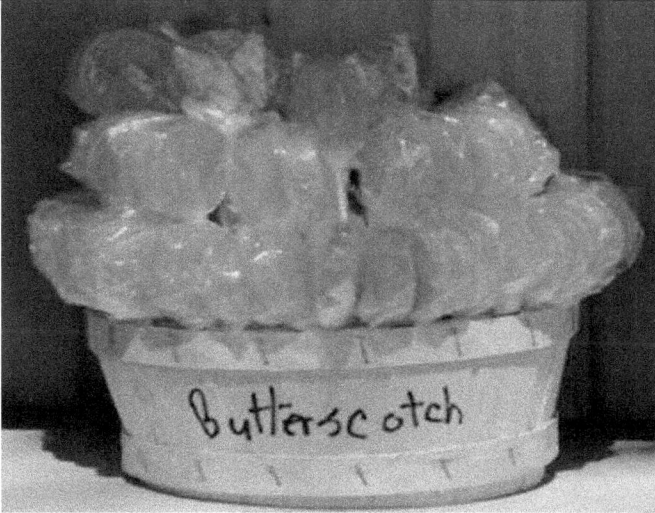

Time Required: 40 Minutes Yield: 12 Cannapops

Ingredients:

1 cup sugar

½ cup cannabis corn syrup 2 tablespoons water

1 ½ teaspoons vinegar

¼ cup cannabutter

¼ teaspoon vanilla extract Lollipop sticks

Directions:

1.   Line baking sheet with waxed paper; set aside. Use cannabutter to grease the sides of the saucepan.

2.   Combine the sugar, cannabis corn syrup, water and vinegar. Cook over medium-high heat for about 5 minutes to boiling, stirring constantly with a wooden spoon to dissolve the sugar. Continue to cook the mixture over medium heat, stirring

constantly, while adding the butter (cut into 8 pieces), 2 pieces at a time.

3.   The candy mixture should boil at a moderate, steady rate over the entire surface. Wait for a candy thermometer to read 300 degrees. This should take 25 to 30 minutes.

4.   Remove the saucepan from the heat. Stir in the vanilla extract. Cool for 5 minutes.

5.   Pour the mixture, 1 to 2 tablespoons at a time, onto the lined baking sheets. The mixture will make 2 to 3 inch circles.

6.   Quickly place a lollipop stick into each piece of candy, twisting gently to cover with the candy mixture. Let the lollipops harden. Wrap the lollipops individually in clear plastic wrap to store at room temperature.

78. Cannabis Hard Candy

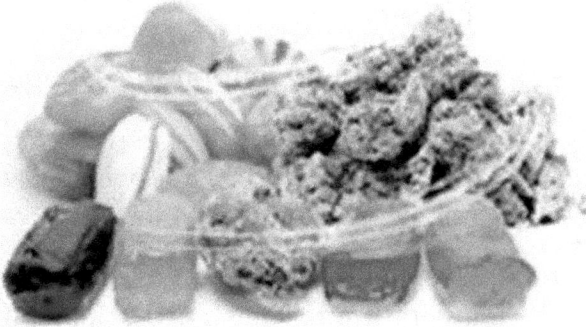

Cannabis hard candy is not only delicious, but holds many benefits for medical users. The amount of THC/CBD in each candy can be measured with precision, and they're easy to eat, especially for people with throat or mouth issues. This recipe will walk you through how to create a whole tray of weed candy for you and your loved ones!

Ingredients:

1 cup cannabutter 2 cups white sugar

¾ cup water

¼ cup honey

½ cup corn or rice syrup

½ teaspoon sea salt

1   teaspoon vanilla or almond extract

2   tablespoons regular butter or coconut oil

Directions:

1.   Heat your honey and cannabutter to the point that they're in a liquid, pourable state. Set aside.

2.   Use the regular butter or coconut oil to coat your candy molds.

3.   Heat sugar, water and corn/rice syrup in a saucepan. Cover without stirring and bring to a boil.

4.   Once the mixture is boiling, use a candy thermometer to check heat until the temperature reaches 132°C, the "soft-crack" stage. This should take about 15 minutes past the point of boiling.

5.   Stir in cannabutter, salt and honey and continue heating until the mixture reaches 148°C. This is the "hard-crack" stage, and now the mixture should bubble to the edges of the pot.

6.   Turn off the heat, wait for the bubbles to subside, and stir in the vanilla or almond extract.

7.   Pour the mixture into the molds. If you're using lollipop sticks, place one end in the mold with the candy.

8.   Allow the candy to cool for 30–60 minutes. Press the candy out of the molds afterwards.

9.   Wrap the candy in aluminum foil or wax paper and refrigerate.

N.B. Remember that edibles can hit harder then you expect, so feel free to judge the amount of cannabis you use to make the butter according to your own experience.

79. Pina Co-Canna Pie Cake

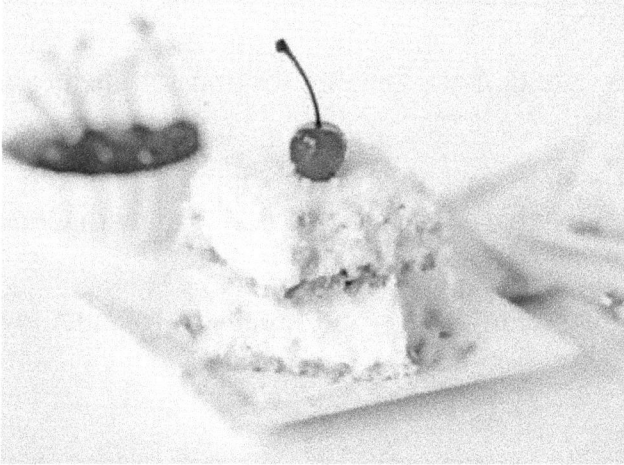

Time Required: 2 hours 30 minutes Yield: 20 pieces

Ingredients:

1½ cups Graham crackers, crumbled

½ cup cannabutter, softened

16 ounces (2- 8 ounce packages) cream cheese, softened

½ cup cream of coconut

½ cup Cool Whip

½ cup pineapple, crushed diced

½ cup cherries, diced

1 cup coconut, shredded

Directions:

1.   Mix graham cracker crumbs and softened cannabutter in a large bowl.

2.   Transfer crust mixture to 9x13 inch baking pan. Press down firmly to cover surface of baking pan with Graham cracker mixture.

3.   Beat cream cheese and cream of coconut together until smooth.

4.   Add cool whip, pineapple and cherries. Fold ingredients together until evenly mixed.

5.   Spread filling mixture on top of the Graham cracker crust. Top with shredded coconut.

6.   Chill cake in refrigerator for 2 hours. Serve and enjoy.

80.   Red-Hot White Fudge

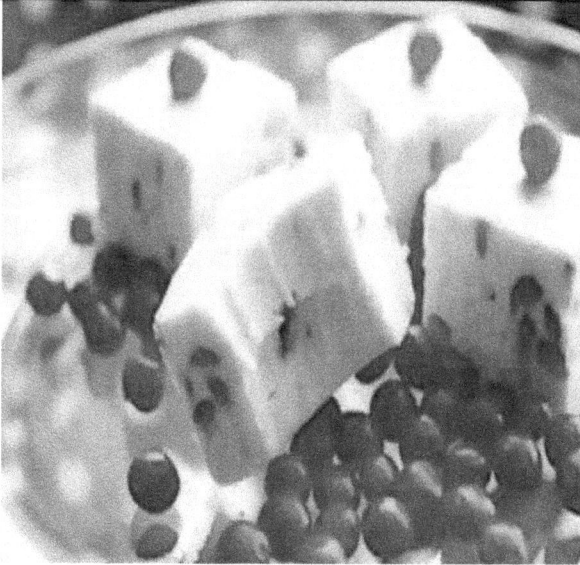

Try something new with this spicy, creamy white fudge. This medicated recipe features a traditional white fudge made with cinnamon oil and and decorated with cinnamon candies to give this treat a kick! Spice up your taste buds with this dreamy, delectable dessert.

Yield: 12-15 Pieces

Ingredients:

1   (14 oz) can sweetened condensed milk 12 ounce bag of white chocolate chips

2-4   ounce baking bars Ghirardelli white chocolate

2   jars red hot cinnamon candies (i.e. Red Hots or Cake Mate cinnamon decors)

12-14 drops cinnamon flavoring oil

2 tablespoons cannabis-infused coconut oil (melted)

Directions:

1.	Line an 8×8 inch pan with wax paper, making sure that the wax paper covers all the way up the sides of the pan.

2.	Pour the sweetened condensed milk into a medium-size sauce pan.

3.	Grab the white chocolate chips and break up the white chocolate bars; add them both to the condensed milk in your sauce pan.

4.	Place the sauce pan over medium-low heat on your stove top, and melt the 3 ingredients together until the chocolate and milk are smooth.

5.	Once the ingredients are creamy and smooth, add the 2 tablespoons of cannabis-infused coconut oil, and mix until the oil is fully combined with the chocolate. (The coconut oil will add a nice sheen to the fudge, too!)

6.	After the coconut oil is combined, remove the sauce pan from the heat.

7.	Stir in the 12-14 drops of cinnamon oil, tasting the chocolate afterwards and adjusting if you desire more spice. (Keep in mind you will also be adding the cinnamon candies).

8.	Add 1½ bottles of your cinnamon candies. (You will be using the remaining ½ bottle of candies to decorate the tops of your white fudge.)

9.	Once the candies are mixed in, pour the white fudge batter into your prepped baking dish, spreading the fudge out with a spatula to ensure a smooth top and filled-in corners.

10.	Place the remaining cinnamon candies on top of the fudge while trying to keep in mind how you will be slicing up the fudge. (I recommend standard rectangle pieces.)

11.   Place the white fudge into the refrigerator, and chill the fudge for at least 2-3 hours or until firm.

12.   Remove the white fudge from the refrigerator, and carefully lift the sides of the wax paper to remove it from the pan. Carefully remove the wax paper from the fudge itself.

13.   If you are giving the fudge as a gift, I suggest you cut off the edge pieces, as they will appear to be a little wrinkled in appearance. Nonetheless, they are still delicious!

14.   Proceed to cut the cinnamon white fudge into pieces that fit your liking.

15.   Serve immediately and enjoy! You can store the fudge pieces in the refrigerator for up to one week.

www.ingramcontent.com/pod-product-compliance
Lightning Source LLC
Chambersburg PA
CBHW050723030426
42336CB00012B/1386